Infectious
Diseases

Infectious Diseases

by

Philip D. Welsby

Consultant Physician
Infectious Diseases Unit
City Hospital
Edinburgh

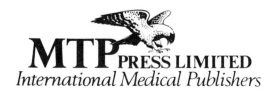

MTP PRESS LIMITED
International Medical Publishers

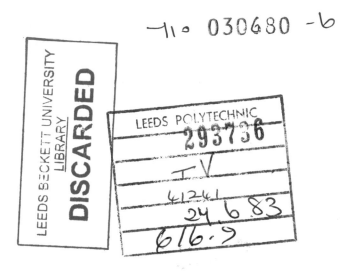
Published by
MTP Press Limited
Falcon House
Lancaster, England

Copyright © 1981 P. D. Welsby

First published 1981

ISBN 0 85200−385−4

Phototypesetting by Swiftpages Ltd., Liverpool
Printed and Bound in Great Britain by
Butler & Tanner Ltd., Frome and London

Contents

Contents

Contents

Introduction

Traditionally only those physicians with many years of experience in a particular speciality chose to commit their accumulated knowledge to print for general consumption. Although of relatively tender years I can remember and sympathize with the problems of learning the 'Infectious Disease Trade' as a medical student and later as a junior hospital doctor. This book is an attempt to journey through and remedy my ignorance-in-retrospect. I have thus attempted to provide an unashamedly clinical introduction to Infectious Diseases which is of particular interest and use to medical students and junior hospital staff, especially those about to enter General Practice.

I hope I have succeeded.

Suggested further reading

Christie, A.B. (1974). *Infectious Diseases: Epidemiology and Clinical Practice.* (Edinburgh: Churchill Livingstone)

Hoeprich, P.D. (1977). *Infectious Diseases.* (London: Harper and Row)

Ramsay, A.M. and Emond, R.T.D. (1978). *Infectious Diseases.* (London: Heinemann Medical Books)

Youmans, G.P., Paterson, P.Y. and Sommers, H.M. (1975). *The Biologic and Clinical Basis of Infectious Disease.* (W.B. Saunders Company)

1
Infection and infectious diseases: basic principles

INTRODUCTION

Infection may be defined as an abnormal state caused by multiplication of pathogenic microorganisms in or on the body of a host: this may cause disease, have no observable effect, or may even be of benefit to an infected host. In common usage, an infection is an infectious disease if the infection is liable to be transmitted such that appropriate isolation of the patient may be required. Put another way, every patient with an infectious disease has an infection, but not all infected patients have an infectious disease.

Fever is an accompaniment to most significantly invasive infections whatever the nature of the causative organism. However, a lack of febrile response to infection may occur in the very young, the very old and the very ill. This febrile response to most infections is caused by a common mediator, endogenous pyrogen, produced by phagocytic leukocytes in response to exogenous pyrogens derived from organisms or their toxic or immunologically active products. Endogenous pyrogen is also produced by hepatic Kupffer cells, splenic sinusoidal cells, alveolar macrophages and peritoneal lining cells — explaining the febrile response to infection by patients who have few or no leukocytes in their blood. The endogenous pyrogen causes fever by resetting the temperature regulating centre in the hypothalamus, possibly by causing increased production of prostaglandins, monoamines and cyclic adenosine monophosphate. The temperature regulating centre then initiates an increase in body temperature, predominantly by acting upon the vasomotor centre which alters peripheral blood flow, thereby regulating heat loss.

Several interesting features arise which can be explained by these mechanisms:

(1)   In febrile patients the temperature regulating centre can be considered to be set at a higher level than normal with a result that the patient may complain of feeling cold (when actually hot) and indeed may undertake violent physical exertion in the form of shivering or a rigor, in order to raise his temperature.

(2)   Aspirin and related drugs possibly reduce fever by interference with prostaglandin synthesis in the hypothalamus.

(3)   Maximum fever may occur *after* the invasion of the blood by bacteria, because there is a delay before blood leukocytes react and liberate endogenous pyrogen: thus blood cultures are probably better taken as the temperature is rising rather than after the peak of the fever.

The pattern of a fever seems to reflect the nature of the infection without being characteristic of any one causative organism. *A remittent fever* is a persisting swinging temperature which varies by one degree centigrade or more and which is elevated for the whole, or almost the whole, of the day. This pattern is found in most infections and presumably reflects the varying progress of the host versus invading pathogen battle. *An intermittent fever* consists of abrupt episodes of fever with return to normal. This pattern may be seen in infections in which intermittent showers of organisms are released – such as occurs in malaria if it is left untreated. *A continued fever* consists of a persistently raised temperature, suggesting a continuously active process such as acute infective endocarditis, or other conditions giving rise to chronic infection of the bloodstream. *An undulant fever* is a fever in which there are periods of fever usually lasting for days, separated by afebrile periods often lasting for weeks rather than days, the pattern presumably reflecting the cyclical nature of some infections – brucella infections may exhibit this pattern.

No matter what the cause, infection related fever may be accompanied by malaise, nausea, headache, vague muscle ache, vasoconstriction, shivering or rigors.

CRITERIA OF PATHOGENICITY

Potentially pathogenic organisms must be able to fulfil certain criteria before they can be successful in producing disease.

(1)   The organism must be able to arrive at the host by a suitable route. *Aerosol or droplet spread* is most suitable for small lightweight

organisms such as viruses, as this mode of spread enables them to achieve widespread dissemination in the environment. *Direct contact, mechanical means or fomite transmission* is more suitable for heavier organisms including most bacteria. *Transmission by a vector* (a living carrier of infection from one organism to another) is necessary if the transmitted organism is incapable of surviving outside a host. For example, most typhus infections require insect vectors for transmission to man. *Transplacental spread* is an important mode of spread for certain infections: the foetus has many vulnerable developing organs and its defences are insufficiently developed to eradicate some infections. Some transplacentally acquired infections such as rubella may persist (with chronic excretion) until well after birth. *Iatrogenic transmission* occurs if doctors unknowingly give infected products to patients, for example bacterially contaminated infusions or blood derived products containing hepatitis B virus.

(2) The infecting organisms have to adhere to appropriate body surfaces and often their adherence capacity is limited to certain tissues: for example shigella bacteria adhere preferentially to intestinal cells whereas influenza viruses adhere preferentially to respiratory tract epithelium.

(3) Subsequently pathogenic organisms pass through an intermediate stage of *colonization* (in which growth is restricted to host surfaces) leading to establishment of the infection.

(4) The infecting organisms are now in a position to attack the host: injury is produced by local or general spread, production of injurious substances, competition with the host for vital nutrients, release of inflammatory substances, production of damage by pressure or obstruction, stimulation of immune responses, or by interference with phagocytosis or phagocytic killing.

Whether or not an illness results from infection usually depends on the interaction between the particular invading organism and the host's defences. In patients with impaired responses to infection (such as the malnourished or the immunosuppressed) the normally harmless indigenous human bacterial flora may be able to realize their latent invasive potential: leukaemic patients are thus vulnerable to invasion by their resident bacteria.

THE HOST'S NATURAL DEFENCES (Figure 1)

Non-specific defences

Non-specific defences against infection include bodily secretions, alterations in the circulating white cell count, local inflammatory responses

IMMUNE SYSTEM
(slower on first challenge to antigens but a more
specific second line of defence)

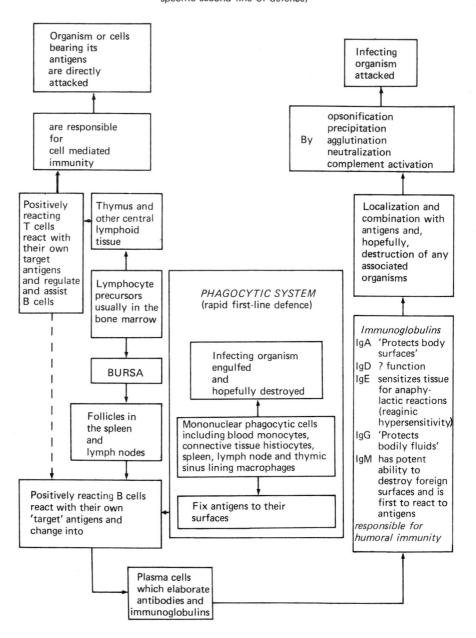

Figure 1   The host's defences against infection or antigenic challenge

and the ingestion of infecting organisms by polymorphonuclear leukocytes and macrophages (the latter include monocytes and reticuloendothelial system cells). These defence mechanisms can react very rapidly to infection.

Specific defences

Specific defences depend substantially on the immune system which, in vertebrates at least, appears to have developed as a defence against infection or internal neoplasia. The immune system reacts slowly to the first challenge with a particular infecting organism, its antigens or toxic products. Selected clones of lymphocytes multiply in response to the infecting agent. The B lymphocytes react and turn into plasma cells and produce antibodies*. The B lymphocytes are assisted and regulated in this by certain thymus derived lymphocytes (T lymphocytes). T lymphocytes are also responsible for cell mediated immunity in which the T lymphocytes act directly against the infecting organism or against the host cell containing them. Cell mediated immunity is often involved in the defence against intracellular infections such as brucellosis or tuberculosis.

The B cells produce five classes of immunoglobulins, nearly all of which are antibodies (the function of some parts of immunoglobulin D is incompletely defined at present).

Immunoglobulin M (IgM)

IgM has potent ability to destroy foreign surface proteins and, presumably as the surface of an infecting agent is the first part of the agent to present itself to the host defence, IgM is the first to increase in an infection: it tends to fade rapidly as the other immunoglobulin classes (particularly IgG) increase. Thus a raised *total* IgM provides strong circumstantial evidence of a recent infection, and if an *organism specific* IgM is raised the evidence of an acute infection with that organism is overwhelming.

Immunoglobulin G (IgG)

IgG 'protects bodily fluids' and usually increases later than IgM (as if to restrain generalized spread of infection after the local battle at the site of invasion). After a specific infection the *organism specific* IgG tends to remain at an increased level and at a (usually) much higher level if there is an active chronic infection.

---

*Antibody may be defined as an immunoglobulin synthesized in response to a specific antigen, an antigen being a substance which elicits the formation of an antibody. All antibodies are immunoglobulins but not all immunoglobulins are definitely known to be antibodies.

Immunoglobulin A (IgA)

IgA 'protects the body surfaces'. It is often found in mucosal surfaces, such as the gut and nasal passages, providing local immunity to infection.

Immunoglobulin E (IgE)

IgE is notably involved in anaphylactic reactions which seem to play little part in the pathogenesis of most infections. IgE is often raised in worm infections, particularly in those which have an extra-intestinal pattern of host invasion.

These immunoglobulins can localize and combine with foreign antigens, hopefully assisting or initiating destruction of the associated invading organisms. In addition various antigen–antibody interactions can activate the complement cascade which results in cell destruction as cell walls are 'physiologically perforated'.

Infection with a specific organism gives rise to an increase in the *organism specific* immunoglobulins of various classes and these rises may be responsible for rises of *total* immunoglobulin. For example, a large rise in *Brucella specific* IgM may cause the *total* serum IgM to be raised. Measurement of *total* immunoglobulin may not be useful in a particular infection if the increase in *organism specific* immunoglobulin does not increase the total quantity of immunoglobulin above normal: it is thus fortunate that modern techniques allow quantification of *organism specific* immunoglobulin responses.

Antigen–antibody reactions are grouped into three main categories (Figure 2), T lymphocyte mediated immunity forms a fourth category in which the T lymphocytes attack cells directly. A fifth category of immunity occurs when antibody stimulates endocrine cells by acting on surface receptors.

Natural active immunity

Natural active immunity is immunity gained by exposure to organisms, their antigens or their toxins: in a previously unprepared host immunity develops slowly (usually taking at least 7 days) but in general active immunity persists for years. Previous exposure to live or dead organisms, their antigens, weakened (attenuated) strains of the natural infection, or other organisms with similar antigens may greatly enhance antibody response to subsequent infections as well as providing 'waiting' antibody.

Natural passive immunity

Natural passive immunity is gained by transplacental transfer of IgG which gives a baby about 6 months protection from most, but not all, infectious diseases to which the mother has antibodies.

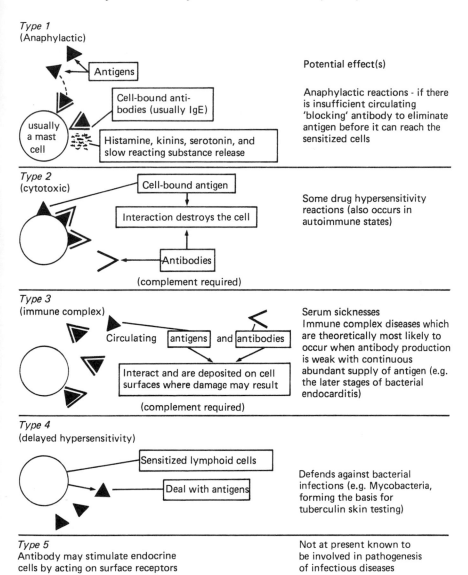

Type 1
(Anaphylactic)

Antigens

Cell-bound anti-bodies (usually IgE)

usually a mast cell

Histamine, kinins, serotonin, and slow reacting substance release

Type 2
(cytotoxic)

Cell-bound antigen

Interaction destroys the cell

Antibodies

(complement required)

Type 3
(immune complex)

Circulating antigens and antibodies

Interact and are deposited on cell surfaces where damage may result

(complement required)

Type 4
(delayed hypersensitivity)

Sensitized lymphoid cells

Deal with antigens

Type 5
Antibody may stimulate endocrine cells by acting on surface receptors

Potential effect(s)

Anaphylactic reactions - if there is insufficient circulating 'blocking' antibody to eliminate antigen before it can reach the sensitized cells

Some drug hypersensitivity reactions (also occurs in autoimmune states)

Serum sicknesses
Immune complex diseases which are theoretically most likely to occur when antibody production is weak with continuous abundant supply of antigen (e.g. the later stages of bacterial endocarditis)

Defends against bacterial infections (e.g. Mycobacteria, forming the basis for tuberculin skin testing)

Not at present known to be involved in pathogenesis of infectious diseases

Figure 2   A classification of immune responses. (Adapted from *Update*)

In summary there is, in most invasive infections, a rapid first-line defence by the phagocytic system: this response merges and integrates with the later, but more specific, immune system responses. In addition, complement activation may occur. However the immune system and immunoglobulin production do not seem to play a part in the recovery from many transitory infections as clinical recovery often occurs too soon for reactive antibody to be responsible.

9

DIAGNOSIS OF INFECTION

Certain infections may present with diagnostic clinical features such that confirmation of the organism responsible is hardly necessary: on occasion a clinical diagnosis allows treatment without the need for laboratory sensitivity tests (for example erysipelas always responds to penicillin).

Rapid confirmation of infection

Rapid confirmation of infection may be achieved by microscopic visualization of the organism, utilizing various stains where appropriate. Microscopy of infected material may reveal changes suggestive of infection with particular organisms even though the organisms themselves cannot be seen. Electron microscopy of infected material may reveal virus particles which may have a diagnostic appearance.

Exposure of an organism or its antigens to antibody (labelled with a fluorescent compound) will result in antigen–antibody interaction, such that some labelled antibody will remain attached after the preparation has been washed. If fluorescence then occurs on exposure to ultraviolet light, one can then confirm that an antigen–antibody interaction had occurred, and thus the associated organism must have been present.

In certain infections other means may exist to make a rapid diagnosis. For example counter current immunoelectrophoresis can be performed on various bodily fluids to identify and differentiate between antigenic patterns of likely pathogens: the cerebrospinal fluid in bacterial meningitis may contain antigens of the causative bacteria even if Gram stain and culture are unhelpful.

Less rapid confirmation of infection

Even if an organism can be cultured, its growth may take time (weeks in tuberculosis for example). Organisms may also be cultured in the presence of various therapeutic agents: differential growth patterns may identify the particular organism and provide therapeutically useful sensitivity results.

Infection with certain organisms can be confirmed (usually in retrospect) by demonstrating changing concentrations (titres) of organism specific antibody in serum samples collected at an interval of at least 1 week (paired sera): ideally such tests should be performed on the two samples simultaneously to minimize experimental errors. Such tests include measurement of the serum's capacity to neutralize laboratory organisms, or to agglutinate appropriately prepared blood cells, or to combine with laboratory prepared antigen with the consumption of complement (complement fixation tests). These tests have a shared basic principle –

that a laboratory preparation of an organism plus the serum (which contained a sufficient amount of antibody against that organism) will elicit an effect not produced by a laboratory preparation of the organism plus serum not containing the antibody. In complement fixation tests the antigen–antibody reaction is detected by complement uptake (complement fixation), which is detected by another complement dependent system (Figure 3). Whichever antibody detecting test is used the

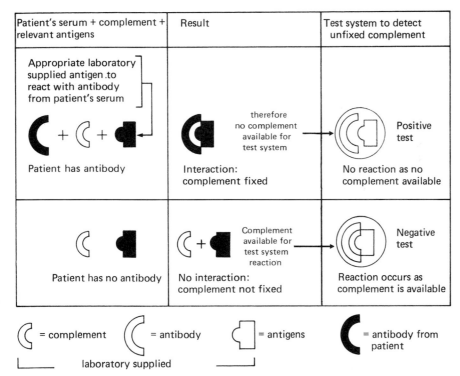

Figure 3   The principle of complement fixation tests. Complement is a substance used up in some antigen–antibody interactions: the fixation of complement by the patient's serum plus laboratory antigen system under test is usually demonstrated by failure of lysis of erythrocytes mixed with erythrocyte antibody–which also requires complement

amount of antibody can be measured by progressively diluting the patient's serum and noting the dilution at which the initial effect fails to be produced. For each serum of a pair, serial dilutions in successive test tubes are used to give dilution ratios 1:1, 1:2, 1:4, 1:8, 1:16, etc. A one tube difference in antibody titre between two paired sera may be difficult to interpret especially if the reaction is borderline: an unequivocal change usually requires at least a two tube difference in antibody concentration between two paired sera (i.e. at least a four-fold change in antibody titre).

11

However, if there is a single high titre of specific antibody to a particular organism this may provide strong circumstantial evidence of an infection with that organism — especially if the presence (or the titre) of the antibody were unusual for the patient's population group. If a patient has been ill for longer than one week before presentation the antibody titres in the first specimen of serum may be diagnostically significant.

Metabolic tests on infected cells may reveal evidence of dysfunction diagnostic of certain infections.

Skin tests can be used to measure skin based reactivity (not necessarily immunity) to various organisms, their antigens or their toxins.

INFECTION AND THE BLOOD

Infection often produces changes in the blood and simple investigations of diagnostic importance can often be performed with relative ease and rapidity.

Anaemia

Infection related anaemia is often multifactorial in origin. Haemorrhage (as may occur in typhoid or hookworm infection), haemolysis (as may occur in malaria or *Clostridium perfringens* infection), or bone marrow depression may each play a part. Mild infections in otherwise healthy patients rarely cause anaemia. Severe acute infections or chronic infections may each produce anaemia in which the circulating erythrocytes are of normal colour and size (normochromic and normocytic). If infection is severe and protracted the erythrocytes may come to contain less haemoglobin (hypochromia) and may also become smaller than normal (microcytic). Most anaemias which are caused by infection rarely respond to iron or vitamin supplements until the infection is controlled: blood transfusions will only provide temporary support. Very rarely certain infections can cause total failure of blood production — aplastic anaemia.

Haemolytic anaemias (suspected clinically by mild lemon coloured jaundice plus the absence of bile from the urine) may be caused by infections which produce erythrocyte antibodies, or which attack the erythrocytes from within or without, or which produce mechanical lesions (endocarditic heart valves for example, which cause haemolysis because of gross turbulence of blood flow).

The erythrocyte sedimentation rate (ESR)

Elevation of the ESR is usually produced by increased fibrinogen production by the liver, or by increased plasma protein constituents (particularly antibodies) or by damage to the erythrocytes, or by a combination of these causes. Each of these causes may result in red cell aggregation or rouleaux formation, which initiates an excessive rate of fall of the erythrocytes in the column of blood in an ESR tube. Interestingly, sickle cells (naturally occurring deformed red blood cells), which cannot form rouleaux successfully, may be associated with absent or minimal elevation of the ESR in conditions which would normally be associated with an elevated ESR.

In most uncomplicated viral infections (such as the common cold) the ESR is normal or only minimally raised, whereas in most invasive bacterial infections the ESR is elevated unless the infection is overwhelming – when the ESR may be low.

Extremely high ESRs, more than 90 mm/hour, when caused by an abrupt recent onset infection, should raise the possibility of mycoplasma infection (in which specific cold agglutinins may initiate the ESR rise) or septicaemia.

The peripheral blood white cell response to infection

Polymorphonuclear leukocytes are motile and can ingest and kill most small infecting agents including most bacteria: however, some organisms may survive and indeed prosper in this intracellular environment. A *leukocytosis* (more than 10.0×10^9 cells/litre) generally reflects an increased demand for white cells to combat infections – which are often bacterial in aetiology. In some severe bacterial infections (staphylococcal septicaemia for example) leukocyte production may fall due to bone marrow depression. *Leukopenia* (less than 4.0×10^9 cells/litre) is classically associated with viral infections and some chronic bacterial infections such as typhoid or tuberculosis: the leukopenia is often caused by a reduction in the neutrophils. A *shift to the left* reflects the varying distribution of certain leukocytes when blood is being smeared across a slide during the preparation of a blood film. It reflects the number of mono- and bi-lobed forms present and is often proportional to the 'clinical toxaemia'.

A *lymphocytosis* (more than 4.0×10^9 cells/litre) often occurs in response to viral infections and reflects an increased demand for both T and B lymphocytes. Viral infections and certain non-viral intracellular infections are often controlled or eliminated by the integrated actions of T and B lymphocytes.

When a marked lymphocytosis occurs in glandular fever, cytomegalovirus infection or whooping cough it has to be distinguished from leukaemia – in which there are primitive lymphocytic forms.

Eosinophilia (more than 0.4×10^9 cells/litre) is often found when there are antigen–antibody interactions, when there is sensitization to foreign protein (particularly worm infections) or in drug allergy reactions – indeed the presence of eosinophilia would provide strong support for either of the latter two diagnoses. An *eosinopenia* often accompanies acute bacterial infections and the return of the eosinophil count to normal may reflect impending recovery from a bacterial infection.

ISOLATION OF PATIENTS

Isolation techniques may be used to protect vulnerable patients, their medical or nursing attendants, or the community. Patients who are excreting transmissible pathogens can be isolated, with appropriate precautions, to prevent spread of infection *to contacts* (barrier nursing), whereas patients who are particularly vulnerable to infection can be isolated *to protect them* from environmental pathogens (reverse barrier nursing).

Patients with the common uncomplicated infectious diseases may be kept at home until the period of infectivity is over, if the home circumstances are suitable. Table 1 details some common infectious diseases which can usually be managed at home and the precautions that should be taken. Isolation from other susceptibles in the home is usually impractical and in any case the susceptibles will often have been most exposed before the diagnosis has been made. However, it may be possible to anticipate the development of certain illnesses in contacts and to isolate them for *their* predicted period of infectivity. Bed linen and pyjamas should ideally be washed at home when fomites are a possible means of transmission.

Table 1 Infectious disease precautions to be taken in some common infectious diseases which can be managed at home

Disease	Precautions
Chickenpox	—
Infective hepatitis A diarrhoea	Spread of infection by faecal–oral route. If possible patients should have the use of their own toilet, they should wash their hands frequently and should not prepare food for others
Hepatitis B	Patients should be made aware, but not unduly terrified by, the potential infectivity of blood, and all other bodily fluids and excreta
Infectious mononucleosis	—
Mumps	—
Rubella	Ensure that there has not been, and will not be, any contact with pregnant women

Patients who should be admitted to infectious disease units include:

(1) Infected patients who are a danger to the community, including carriers of certain infections and patients on general hospital wards who are excreting highly resistant organisms.

14

(2) Patients who are in unsatisfactory circumstances for management of their infection – the socially deprived, travellers, students, children in nurseries, the homeless and those resident in hotels.
(3) Seriously ill patients who have, or may have, an infectious disease.
(4) Patients who require safe investigation of pyrexias of unknown origin, febrile rashes or diarrhoeal illnesses.

Suggested further reading

Myrvik, Q.N., Pearsall, N.N. and Russell, S.W. (1974). *Fundamentals of Medical Bacteriology and Mycology*. (Philadelphia: Lea and Febiger)

Playfair, J.H.L. (1979). *Immunology at a Glance*. (Oxford: Blackwell Scientific Publications)

Jamieson, J.R. (1977). *Man meets Microbes*. (Sevenoaks: Butterworths)

Mims, C.A. (1977). *The Pathogenesis of Infectious Disease*. (London: Academic Press)

2
Bacterial infections

An understanding of bacterial structure is essential for the understanding of pathogenic mechanisms (Figure 4).

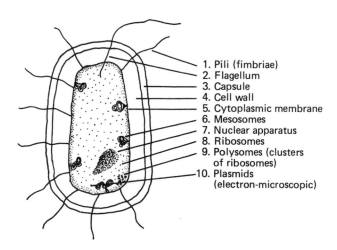

1. Pili (fimbriae)
2. Flagellum
3. Capsule
4. Cell wall
5. Cytoplasmic membrane
6. Mesosomes
7. Nuclear apparatus
8. Ribosomes
9. Polysomes (clusters of ribosomes)
10. Plasmids (electron-microscopic)

Figure 4   The possible anatomical features of bacteria

Pili (also known as fimbriae) are of two types. Holdfast pili are usually found in gram-negative bacteria such as the gonococcus, *Proteus* sp., *Pseudomonas* sp., *Salmonella* sp. and *Shigella* sp. enabling them to adhere to various host surfaces whereas sexual pili can transfer genetic information to other bacteria, including information for drug resistance.

Flagellae give their possessors mobility.

The capsule is an outer 'slime' layer which can protect against phagocytic attack.

Bacterial cell walls are composed of various layers. Cell wall uptake of Gram's stain reflects the physical properties of the cell wall and pathogenic potential of the bacteria: gram-positive bacteria have a relatively simple cell wall whereas gram-negative bacteria have numerous, more complex, layers which hinder penetration of antibacterial drugs. The most distinctive cell wall building material is muramic acid and, as mammalian cell walls do not contain this material, its synthesis constitutes a unique biochemical target for certain antibacterial drugs such as penicillin or the cephalosporins. However some bacteria may be intrinsically resistant to these drugs, other bacteria may produce specific enzymes which destroy the drug, and other bacteria can temporarily abandon their vulnerable cell wall (forming the so-called L forms) whilst under drug attack and are thus enabled to persist.

The cytoplasmic membranes maintain the bacterial intracellular environment, act as an osmotic barrier, and indirectly synthesize the bacterial cell wall. Mesosomes are invaginations of the cytoplasmic membrane which produce energy in a manner somewhat analogous to mammalian mitochondria.

Ribosomes are the sites of protein synthesis and are relatively vulnerable to drugs such as streptomycin.

Plasmids are genetic elements which only exist in autonomous forms and which are not known to be capable of integrating with bacterial chromosomes. They can be transmitted to other bacteria, possibly conferring pathogenically useful information (such as the information required to produce drug resistance).

Some bacteria, notably *Bacillus anthracis* and the Clostridia can form spores which are extremely resistant survival vehicles and which can later give rise to the parent bacteria when suitable conditions arise. Spores require autoclaving* for eradication.

Various bacterial structures, particularly the external pili, flagella and capsule, may elicit antibody production by an invaded host.

In addition to the previously mentioned general methods of attack bacteria may produce toxins, of which there are two groups. *Exotoxins* are

---

*Autoclaving is the utilization of steam under temperature in excess of 100 °C using appropriate pressures for minimum specified times.

usually liberated by live gram-positive bacteria. They are strongly anti-genic, highly toxic towards specific tissues, easily converted to toxoids† and readily neutralized by antibodies. In contrast, *endotoxins* are released when the cell walls (usually of gram-negative bacteria) are disrupted. In general endotoxins are less toxic than exotoxins, not convertible to toxoids, poorly neutralized by antibodies and produce widespread damage to numerous tissues. In theory at least, the initial antibacterial therapy of patients with certain gram-negative septicaemias may increase the endo-toxaemia by disrupting bacteria and their cells walls, thus making the patient worse before making him better.

Some bacteria can exchange potentially pathogenic genetic information by *transformation* in which segments of bacterial DNA enter other bacteria, *transduction* in which certain bacterial viruses (phages) transport genetic information from one bacterium to another, and by *conjunction* in which 'male' and 'female' bacteria utilize sexual pili to transfer genetic inform-ation – occasionally a part of a whole 'male' chromosome is transferred.

The bacterial invasion of the host usually elicits a vigorous defensive reaction involving the phagocytes and the immune system (Chapter 1). In addition to these and other defences antibacterial drugs may be prescribed. Presently available drugs have four possible sites of action (Figure 5).

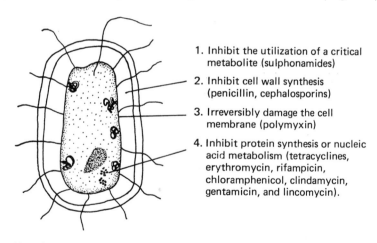

1. Inhibit the utilization of a critical metabolite (sulphonamides)

2. Inhibit cell wall synthesis (penicillin, cephalosporins)

3. Irreversibly damage the cell membrane (polymyxin)

4. Inhibit protein synthesis or nucleic acid metabolism (tetracyclines, erythromycin, rifampicin, chloramphenicol, clindamycin, gentamicin, and lincomycin).

Figure 5   The common sites of attack for antibacterial drugs

When clinical symptoms or signs of a particular disease commence the incubation period is over and a working diagnosis must be made: 'informed guess' therapy may be indicated after appropriate specimens have been obtained to (hopefully) confirm the diagnosis.

---

†A toxoid is a toxin treated to destroy its deleterious properties without destroying its ability to stimulate antibody production.

In theory at least, antibacterial drugs can be divided into two classes, *bacteriostatic* drugs (which prevent bacterial multiplication but which alone do not kill bacteria) and *bactericidal* drugs (which can kill bacteria substantially unassisted by host defences). However, bactericidal drugs given in too low a dosage may be bacteriostatic in action, and the term bacteriostatic often means that one cannot give safely a high enough dose of a drug to result in a bactericidal action. Drugs that have to be used in bacteriostatic fashion usually exert their action on a cellular process that is also present in the host cells, whereas bactericidal drugs (such as penicillins and cephalosporins) often act on structures – such as bacterial cell walls – which are not found in host cells: such drugs are usually less likely to cause serious side effects for the same reason.

Combinations of *two* bacteriostatic drugs (for example co-trimoxazole) may in practice have a bactericidal action with an additional advantage that bacteria, to attain resistance, have to develop simultaneously *two* 'metabolic tricks' – each of which confers resistance to one member of the drug combination.

Bacteriostatic drugs should not be used to treat patients with impaired immune or cellular responses (for example leukaemic or neutropenic patients) as such patients will not be able to destroy the static bacteria – which could restart division after drug withdrawal.

A CLINICALLY BIASED ACCOUNT OF COMMON PATHOGENIC BACTERIA
(Figure 6)

Staphylococcal infections

Staphylococcus epidermis is loosely identical to *Staph. albus* and is a relatively non-pathogenic bacteria, often being found on the human skin as a commensal organism. On occasion it can attack opportunistically, infective endocarditis being the most serious illness produced.

Staph. pyogenes (Staph. aureus). Although often carried by healthy individuals this organism frequently causes severe infections characterized by *localized* lesions such as boils or abscesses, rather than by the spreading infections that streptococci often cause. In general, staphylococci can survive the external environment well and, especially in hospitals, have developed penicillin resistance by the ability to produce penicillinase – a capability which may be transmitted by plasmids.

Minor bloodstream invasion tends to result in focal lesions such as osteo-myelitis or perinephric abscesses. Major invasion produces a septicaemic picture and may also produce an ulcerative endocarditis which can affect previously normal heart valves.

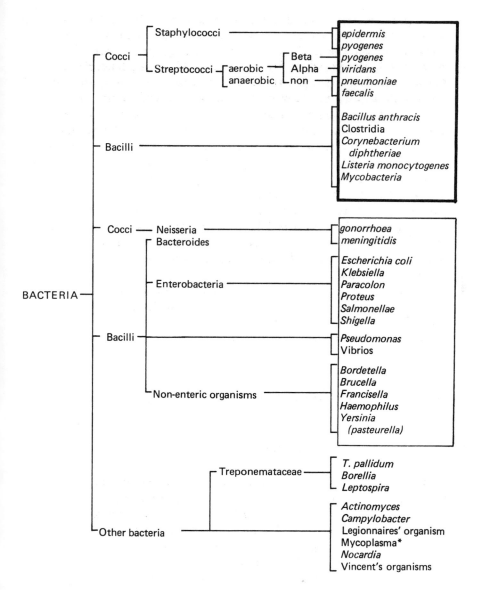

Figure 6   A classification of the major pathogenic bacteria. ☐ = Gram positive; ☐ = Gram negative; * not a true bacteria

Certain strains of staphylococci may cause food poisoning, a condition which classically has an incubation period of less than 6–8 hours and which initially produces vomiting perhaps followed by diarrhoea. Staphylococcal food poisoning is caused by release of a heat resistant toxin which is rapidly absorbed from the gastrointestinal tract and which exerts its action on the central nervous system.

Staphylococcal invasion of the skin may cause a bullous impetigo or, rarely, a toxic epidermal necrolysis – the 'scalded skin' syndrome.

Whenever resistance of staphylococci to penicillin is suspected, drugs such as methicillin or flucloxacillin (which resist the attack of penicillinase) or non-penicillin drugs have to be used. Sensitivity testing is essential as certain staphylococci may be resistant to several drugs. Treatment of asymptomatic carriers of virulent staphylococci with antibacterial drugs is only occasionally successful but can be tried in conjunction with applications of antiseptic solutions.

Streptococcal infections

Streptococci are classified by their ability to haemolyse blood agar. In non-haemolytic strains haemolysis is absent. In α (green)-haemolytic strains there is incomplete haemolysis and in β-haemolysis there is complete haemolysis – a clear region around colonies. β-haemolytic streptococci are classified further into Lancefield *Groups* A, B, C, D etc. according to differences in cell wall *carbohydrate*, and Group A β-haemolytic streptococci (known as *Strep. pyogenes*) are further subdivided into approximately 50 Griffiths *types* depending on cell wall *protein* characteristics.

The spectrum of illnesses produced by streptococcal infection is wide and can be divided approximately into illnesses caused by invasion of the organism into tissues and those illnesses caused by 'immune' mechanisms.

Primarily invasive streptococcal infections

Strep. agalactiae (Lancefield group B) infection is an emerging cause of puerperal fever and neonatal sepsis.

Strep. pyogenes may cause (a) bacterial pharyngitis and tonsillitis: such infections are most common in the 5–15 year age group, and in classical cases there is a severely painful sore throat, without cough or much nasal 'stuffiness' and there may be secondary cervical lymphadenitis. Earache is a common accompaniment. Local extension of infection may lead to quinsy or to retropharyngeal abscess formation. The antistreptolysin O titre (ASOT), an antibody formed as part of the host response, subsequently rises in about 70% of patients. (b) *Impetigo*, if caused by streptococci, classically consists of vesicular or crusted skin lesions. It is readily transmissible, and if extensive, systemic antibacterial therapy is indicated. In clinical situations both staphylococci and streptococci are often isolated and the primary pathogen is uncertain. (c) *Erysipelas* is a streptococcal infection of the skin which usually presents with sudden onset fever in association with a warm, spreading, indurated, erythematous area with well demarcated margins. Erysipelas tends to be a more superficial infection than streptococcal cellulitis: both are usually caused by *Strep. pyogenes* and both invariably respond bacteriologically to penicillin: erythromycin is an alternative therapy in the penicillin allergic patient.

Strep. viridans is a common oral commensal which may cause an infective endocarditis when it alights upon heart valves, especially those previously damaged by an attack of rheumatic fever.

Strep. pneumoniae can be thought of as a predominantly respiratory tract pathogen as it may cause both lobar pneumonia and bronchopneumonia, sinusitis, and otitis media. It may also cause meningitis, particularly after head injury with or without an obvious skull fracture.

Strep. faecalis, also known as the enterococcus, is a possible cause of urinary tract infection and infective endocarditis.

Primarily 'immune-mediated' manifestations of streptococcal infection

Erythema nodosum consists of bruise-like lesions, usually on the shins, which may occur secondary to streptococcal infection, and which are associated with antigen–complement–antibody deposition in blood vessels.

Glomerulonephritis usually occurs 10–20 days after group A streptococcal infections of certain 'nephritogenic' types. It is caused by cross-reactivity or immune complex deposition on the glomerular basement membrane resulting in renal impairment with oliguria, haematuria, proteinuria, oedema and hypertension. Recurrent attacks are rare because of the limited number of nephritogenic strains, because immunity is gained to the strain of the particular organism involved, and because some immunity is also gained by exposure to non-nephritogenic strains of antigenically similar streptococci. Thus long-term prophylaxis with penicillin is rarely indicated.

Henoch–Schönlein (anaphylactoid) purpura often occurs secondary to streptococcal infection which initiates an immune reaction and damages vascular endothelium. There are (Henoch's) purpuric lesions in the skin, particularly over pressure areas, and abdominal and joint pains. Intussusception can occur in young children.

Rheumatic fever may occur 1–4 weeks after group A streptococcal pharyngitis. It is caused by many strains of streptococci and, as recurrences are not unusual, long-term penicillin prophylaxis after one attack is indicated. Rheumatic fever 'licks the joints but bites the heart' and its aetiology hinges on a combination of allergy, cross reactivity and toxic activity of streptococcal constituents. Major diagnostic criteria of rheumatic fever include carditis, arthritis, rheumatoid nodules, chorea or erythema marginatum. Minor criteria include fever, arthralgia, a raised white cell count or ESR, a previous attack of rheumatic fever, delayed atrio-ventricular conduction on electrocardiogram (PR interval prolonged), a raised ASOT, or documented streptococcal pharyngitis. The requirements for a diagnosis of rheumatic fever are two major criteria *or* one major plus two minor criteria *plus* evidence of previous streptococcal infection.

Scarlet fever is uncommon in Britain today. It may occur 2–4 (limits 1–7) days after the start of streptococcal pharyngitis, with sore throat, vomiting, a facial flush with circumoral pallor, a white then red strawberry tongue and a diffuse pink-red cutaneous flush with punctate elements especially noticeable on the abdomen and chest. This scarlet reaction serves as a visible manifestation of a severe streptococcal infection with possible complications including cervical adenitis, otitis media, skin lesions, glomerulonephritis or rheumatic fever. The scarlet rash is caused by an erythrogenic toxin to which immunity is gained and therefore recurrent attacks are unusual.

Sydenham's chorea is generally regarded as a complication of group A streptococcal infection. There are diffuse cerebral changes most marked in the corpus striatum and associated structures.

Bacillus anthracis

This organism forms spores which can remain potentially alive and infectious on soil and other media for decades. Infection occurs by contact with infected animals or their products: human infection is usually occupational and commonly results from spores entering through skin abrasions to cause cutaneous anthrax, or via the respiratory tract to produce a pneumonic illness or an allergic alveolitis. Rarely intestinal anthrax may occur. The hallmark of cutaneous anthrax is the malignant pustule (which is neither a pustule nor malignant). This malignant pustule is classically a solitary, painless, necrotic ulcerated lesion with a black slough (eschar): it may heal spontaneously or serve as an initiating site for septicaemia with associated profound toxaemia. Penicillin or tetracyclines usually result in bacteriological cure but may not cure the toxin mediated component of the illness.

The clostridial species

The pathogenic clostridia secrete highly potent exotoxins and may form highly resistant spores. Anaerobic areas, such as may be found in wounds, intestinal lesions and the uterus, are required to support their growth. Such areas are anaerobic due to lack of blood supply and thus eradication of the organisms by blood-borne therapies alone is unlikely to succeed, and removal or drainage of these anaerobic areas is also required.

Clostridium tetani produces tetanus, the incidence and mortality of which has been greatly reduced by immunization with toxoid which confers immunity to the neurotoxin secreted by this organism. The neurotoxin spreads proximally from the site of infection along motor nerves or via the blood and suppresses inhibitory influences on motor neurones – thereby causing violent painful spasms of voluntary muscles, either localized (as in lockjaw) or generalized. Sympathetic overactivity may cause fever, sweating and cardiovascular problems.

Clostridium perfringens (welchii) is associated with two main illnesses, gas gangrene and food poisoning. Gas gangrene is usually caused by *Clostridium perfringens* but *Cl. oedematiens (novyi)* and *Cl. septicum* may also be responsible. Wound pain and oedema are followed by fever and extreme prostration. Extensive haemolysis associated with leukocytosis and thrombocytopenia may occur especially if septicaemia supervenes. Often fermentation of host tissues causes subcutaneous gas formation recognized clinically by crepitation on digital pressure. The associated tissue swelling may lead to extension of the original ischaemic area resulting in further spread of the anaerobic infection. Treatment depends on surgical intervention up to and including amputation, administration of antibacterial drugs which at least give some protection to contiguous aerobic areas, administration of antitoxin and, if possible, administration of hyperbaric oxygen.

Clostridium perfringens food poisoning occurs within 18 hours of ingestion of an enterotoxin formed when *Cl. perfringens* grows in anaerobic areas within foods.

Clostridium botulinum produces botulism which results from one of six possible neurotoxins produced by various strains of *Cl. botulinum*. The neurotoxins block the release of acetylcholine at cholinergic synapses causing profound paralysis. If death does not occur, neurological recovery usually is complete. Therapy is by urgent administration of antitoxin and management of respiratory muscle paralysis.

Corynebacterium diphtheriae

Diphtheria is a localized infection which causes major neurological and cardiovascular manifestations by means of a powerful slow acting exotoxin. The three main pathogenic strains are named gravis, intermedius and mitis, but the name need not reflect pathogenic potential. Infection is spread by asymptomatic carriers or by a patient with the illness. The organisms are transmitted in droplets which are inhaled and settle on the surface of the nasopharynx, larynx, trachea or oropharynx: they do not invade. During the first week of illness general non-specific symptoms predominate and the course of the following illness depends largely on the site of infection – anterior nasal diphtheria is invariably mild, tonsillar diphtheria intermediate and pharyngeal diphtheria severe. The characteristic membrane (see Chapter 8, page 122) is usually a false membrane in that little epithelium is present. Histologically there is oedema, hyperaemia and a fibrinous exudate which coagulates to form a firmly adherent membrane with epithelial necrosis. Laryngeal diphtheria carries a grave risk of respiratory obstruction.

The effects of the toxin tend to be sequential. In the first week peripheral circulatory failure may occur, and during the second week clinical evidence of heart involvement. If the patient survives this period a predominantly paralytic illness may follow with paralysis, often sequential, of palate, eyes, heart, pharynx and larynx and respiratory muscles with limb paralysis occurring in the seventh to tenth week. The major lesion in the peripheral nerves is demyelination whereas the heart develops a toxic myocarditis and dysrhythmias may occur. Other organs, including the adrenals and kidneys, may also be affected by the toxin.

Listeria monocytogenes

This infection often induces a monocytosis, hence the name. It frequently attacks immunologically vulnerable individuals, including neonates or the elderly, to cause a septicaemia or meningitis. It is sensitive to many antibacterial drugs, including penicillins, tetracyclines, chloramphenicol and erythromycin.

Mycobacterial infections

In Britain tuberculosis is predominantly caused by infection with *Mycobacterium tuberculosis*, which is a weakly gram-positive and obligate aerobic organism. The classical histopathological lesion of tuberculosis is the tubercle (Figure 7).

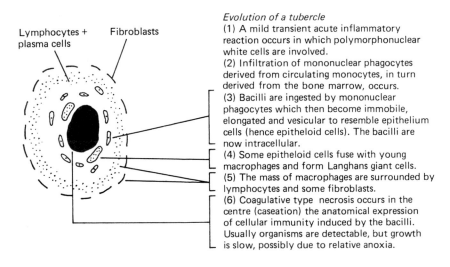

Lymphocytes + plasma cells   Fibroblasts

Evolution of a tubercle
(1) A mild transient acute inflammatory reaction occurs in which polymorphonuclear white cells are involved.
(2) Infiltration of mononuclear phagocytes derived from circulating monocytes, in turn derived from the bone marrow, occurs.
(3) Bacilli are ingested by mononuclear phagocytes which then become immobile, elongated and vesicular to resemble epithelium cells (hence epitheloid cells). The bacilli are now intracellular.
(4) Some epitheloid cells fuse with young macrophages and form Langhans giant cells.
(5) The mass of macrophages are surrounded by lymphocytes and some fibroblasts.
(6) Coagulative type necrosis occurs in the centre (caseation) the anatomical expression of cellular immunity induced by the bacilli. Usually organisms are detectable, but growth is slow, possibly due to relative anoxia.

Figure 7   Tubercle formation

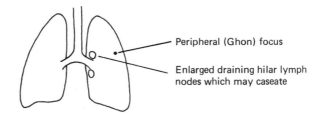

Usually occurs in lung

Peripheral (Ghon) focus

Enlarged draining hilar lymph
nodes which may caseate

Figure 8   Initial exposure (primary complex) tuberculosis. There is essentially unrestricted local growth, both extra- and intracellularly. Spread may occur before acquired immunity and/or hypersensitivity occurs, especially in the very young, very old and the immunocompromised. The primary focus can occur anywhere, e.g. in the pharynx (especially in *Myco. bovis* infection) with neck glands, in the bowel with mesenteric adenopathy, and in the skin after BCG vaccination

Primary complex infection (Figure 8)

Primary complex infection occurs after first infection with *Mycobacterium tuberculosis* and usually occurs in the lungs.

There may be three outcomes of primary complex tuberculosis:

(1)   The tuberculous lesions may proliferate and then heal because of a granulomatous reaction with associated fibrosis and calcification.

(2)   The tuberculous lesions may proliferate, soften and caseate, with affected tissues being converted, by degeneration, into an amorphous cheese-like mass.

(3)   An exudative outpouring of fluid may occur because of a marked tissue reaction to the bacilli.

Usually primary complex infections escape notice and heal uneventfully but problems may arise if:

(a)   Viable bacilli persist in healed lesions and later escape to produce secondary complex tuberculosis.

(b)   Infection progresses − progressive primary tuberculosis.

(c)   Distant seeding of bacilli occurs in other organs (such as the adrenals, brain, bone or kidney) and focal pathological effects occur, either at the time or later.

(d)   Generalized miliary spread occurs (without evidence of specific organ involvement).

Secondary complex infection (Figure 9)

Secondary complex infection often occurs in the lungs consequent to a second bout of infection with *Mycobacterium tuberculosis*. These secondary complex bacilli may have escaped from previous primary complexes (probably the most common occurrence) or from inhaled organisms from

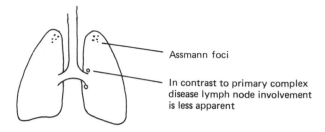

Assmann foci

In contrast to primary complex
disease lymph node involvement
is less apparent

Figure 9   Secondary type complex tuberculosis

the environment. Sometimes it seems that secondary complex tuberculosis
can occur as the result of an initial infection (especially if it occurs in adults
known to be Mantoux negative). There may be three outcomes of secondary complex tuberculosis:

(1)   The complex may heal by fibrosis and/or calcification.
(2)   The Assmann foci may enlarge, soften and caseate, forming
       abscesses which spread locally. Alternatively the abscesses may
       rupture into the airways (tuberculous bronchopneumonia), or may
       rupture or invade the blood or lymphatic vessels – leading to local
       haemorrhage (haemoptysis) or miliary spread of the bacilli.
(3)   Cavity formation occurs if the abscesses drain into the respiratory
       tree: if such cavities are, or become, closed or collapsed (and there-
       fore anaerobic), the contents become thickened and ultimately
       harden and calcify.

If spontaneous or drug assisted healing occurs there may still be dormant
bacilli which may subsequently reactivate.

To diagnose tuberculosis the bacilli have to be seen on a specially stained
smear (Ziehl–Nielsen stain): a routine Gram stain is *most unlikely* to
suggest tuberculous infection. Culture on various media including Lowen-
stein–Jensen medium confirms the diagnosis.

First-line drugs used in the treatment of tuberculosis include isoniazid
(INAH), rifampicin and streptomycin. Other useful drugs include
ethambutol, pyrazinamide, ethionamide, thiacetazone and para-amino-
salicylic acid (PAS). Capreomycin, viomycin and cycloserine are useful but
toxic and are usually only indicated when other drugs are contraindicated
or ineffective. In Britain today the usual initial treatment of pulmonary
tuberculosis is with three drugs, rifampicin, isoniazid and ethambutol.

Ideally patients with pulmonary tuberculosis should be isolated whilst
they are known to be excreting the organisms into the environment. The
evidence available suggests that patients who are receiving treatment but

are smear positive (the stained organisms being visible in the sputum) are more infectious than those who are smear negative, and those who are both smear and culture negative are hardly infectious at all. Opinions differ as to the time at which it is reasonable to relax isolation − it may take 4−8 weeks or longer for a patient to become smear negative. It may also take 6 weeks for cultures to reveal whether patients are still excreting viable tubercle bacilli and whether the bacilli are sensitive to the prescribed drugs.

Leprosy

Mycobacterium leprae infection and the resultant host reaction cause leprosy, in which there is classical involvement of the skin (leading to induration and/or hypopigmentation) and involvement of nervous tissue (leading to altered sensation and nerve thickening). Fortunately transmission usually requires prolonged close contact. If host immunity is strong, *tuberculoid* leprosy results with few organisms demonstrable; but if immunity is weak, *lepromatous* leprosy results with widespread lesions in which the unchecked organisms are frequent. There are intermediate stages.

Neisserial infections

N. gonorrhoeae causes a relatively common illness which is associated with freedom of sexual expression which involve two or more people. The short incubation period (usually 2−8 days), the apparent lack of immunity to reinfection and difficulties in locating and identifying asymptomatic patients (both female and male) all contribute to its perpetuation.

In the male the onset is usually abrupt with painful micturition and urethral discharge. If the infection is confined to the urethra there is no fever, but spread to epididymis, prostate, and bloodstream may cause fever. Most infections in the male would, if untreated, resolve spontaneously but later fibrosis might cause urethral strictures.

In females infection commonly involves the urethra and cervix. Infection may spread to the rectum or Fallopian tubes (salpingitis). Gonorrhoea in females tends to be symptomatically mild in postpubertal females, and persistent low-grade infection may occur. Bloodstream spread occurs occasionally in both sexes with metastatic lesions, peri-hepatitis, dermal lesions, lesions of tendons, joints and heart valves. An allergic arthritis or tenosynovitis may also occur.

Neonatal ophthalmic gonorrhoea can be acquired by the perinate during its passage down the birth canal.

N. meningitidis is commonly spread by asymptomatic carriers and epidemics of meningitis may arise in crowded conditions. The proportion of the normal population that carry the organism in the throat varies between 5% or less and about 20%.

There are three main serogroups, A, B, and C, all of which possess capsules which are important virulence factors and which resist phagocytosis. Endotoxin production probably plays an important part in production of vascular changes.

After an incubation period of 2–3 days the organism passes from the colonized nasopharyngeal mucosa to the central nervous system where it initiates a meningitis. Why it does this in one individual but not in another is substantially unknown. In individuals with an invasive infection a brief or persistent bacteraemia (with or without the development of meningitis) occurs, and a characteristic purpuric rash consisting of small discrete lesions or large irregular blotchy areas (in which the meningococcus is present) may result. Disseminated intravascular coagulation or adrenal haemorrhages may occur in association with severe illnesses: whether the adrenal haemorrhages are only a focal manifestation of the disseminated intravascular coagulation or whether hypoadrenalism contributes significantly are debatable points.

Second attacks are not rare, perhaps suggesting that a particular individual is in some way immunologically vulnerable.

In the past sulphonamides were usually effective but because of the present incidence of sulphonamide resistance, therapy now rests on the urgent intravenous administration of high dose penicillin, with or without sulphonamides. Chloramphenicol is the drug of second choice.

All close contacts should receive prophylactic antibiotic, the choice lying between minocycline or rifampicin: the drug sensitivity of current isolates often determines the drug chosen.

Acinetobacter/Moraxella, perhaps better known as *Mima polymorpha*, can cause a meningitis that mimics meningococcal meningitis. Differentiation is important as both may cause meningitis with a petechial rash, but *Mima polymorpha* is usually resistant to penicillin. This organism is usually sensitive to tetracyclines and kanamycin.

Bacteroides

A large proportion of the human faecal flora are anaerobic gram-negative organisms, mostly bacteroides species. In the normal course of events these remain localized in the bowel. However they may escape, thereby becoming pathogenic, particularly in patients with sepsis after gastrointestinal surgery, patients with malignancies and patients with diabetes mellitus. Possible illnesses produced by bacteroides species include peritonitis, abscesses with characteristically foul smelling pus, necrotizing pneumonias, lung abscesses or brain abscesses. *Bacteroides fragilis* is the most frequent species encountered and it is notable for its resistance to penicillins in the usually administered dosages. The antibacterial drug of choice is probably metronidazole, which has few side effects compared to the other choices which include chloramphenicol, clindamycin or lincomycin. Some recently introduced drugs of the cephalosporin group are also effective.

Escherichia coli

This is a normal resident of the lower gastrointestinal tract and often infects anatomically related areas such as the urinary tract or peritoneum. Certain enterotoxin producing strains are responsible for a proportion of infantile diarrhoea and travellers' diarrhoea. Occasionally non-enterotoxic *E. coli* can produce diarrhoea by invasion of gut epithelium.

E. coli urinary tract infections, as with most other urinary tract infections, are more common in females who lack the long 'protective' urethra of the male. Treatment of urinary infection before receiving microscopy, culture and sensitivity reports must usually assume the presence of *E. coli*.

The most appropriate oral antibacterial drug for *E. coli* urinary tract infections is a matter of debate and often depends on the sensitivity patterns of 'local' *E. coli* isolates. Ampicillin and sulphonamide resistant strains may be a problem: in the presence of renal impairment tetracyclines and nitrofurantoin (although bacteriologically acceptable) should not be used. Co-trimoxazole or cephalosporins are generally effective. Gentamicin and other aminoglycosides have to be given parenterally and because of this are not justified in the majority of infections.

As a general point urinary tract infections in association with anatomical abnormalities (including a urinary catheter) are unlikely to be eliminated by antibacterial therapy.

Escherichia coli may also cause septicaemias, cholecystitis and neonatal meningitis.

Klebsiella

K. pneumoniae (Friedlander's bacillus) is a possible cause of severe pneumonia which on X-ray may show suggestive cavitation and expansion of pneumonic areas (due to extensive oedema). Penicillins are ineffective: possible therapies include the aminoglycosides, co-trimoxazole, tetracyclines, chloramphenicol and cephalosporins. Combination therapy is often utilized.

K. ozaenae causes an offensive nasal discharge with atrophic rhinitis.

K. rhinoscleromatis causes chronic granulomatous lesions of the nose and throat.

Proteus species

These organisms are a frequent cause of urinary tract infections, especially in young boys. All these organisms – *Proteus mirabilis, vulgaris, morgagni* and *rettgeri* – ferment urinary urea and thereby form ammonia, with its characteristic odour. *Proteus mirabilis*, in contrast to the other strains, is usually susceptible to ampicillin.

Recently *P. rettgeri* have been reclassified into the *Providentia* genera and *P. morgagni* into the *Morganella* genera.

Salmonella infections

In general the salmonellae are similar in structure to *E. coli*. They possess various antigens to which antibodies may be formed (Figure 10). A convincing rise in titre of antibody to a particular salmonella organism may be significant but as a screening test for *S. typhi* infection this (Widal) test leaves much to be desired, especially if the patient had previously received TAB vaccination.

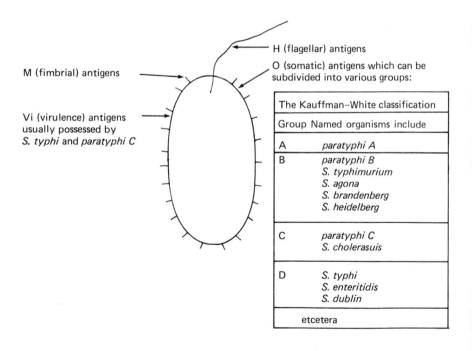

Figure 10   Salmonellae: antigenic classification. The Kauffman–White classification is clinically relevant because the laboratory will often issue a preliminary report of the Group before confirmation of the particular salmonella is known

Salmonellae produce three main clinical illnesses but there may be some overlap.

(1)   The first and commonest type of illness ('gastroenteritis', 'food poisoning'), with diarrhoea and vomiting is produced by infection which usually remains confined to the gut. It may be caused by most of the 1800 or so named salmonella organisms. Relatively large numbers of organisms are required to initiate illness and, as gastric acid provides a protective barrier, patients with low gastric acid levels (post-gastrectomy or in patients with pernicious anaemia) tend to have a more severe illness.

    This type of illness is commonly associated with contaminated foodstuffs and farm products, and farm animals provide a large reservoir of infection. Faulty food preparation is often to blame for human illness because salmonellae can survive freezing, and if carcases thaw the organisms may multiply. If the inner organs of a carcass are incompletely cooked due to their central situation (or because they were still frozen at the start of the cooking) large numbers of surviving salmonellae will be ingested by the recipient of the meal. In the absence of suspected or known bloodstream invasion antibacterial therapy is not indicated in the vast majority of patients with salmonella induced diarrhoea and vomiting.

(2)   The second type of illness is a bacteraemia induced illness with possible focal sepsis in which gastrointestinal symptoms and signs may be minimal or absent. It may be caused by any of the salmonellae.

(3)   The third type of illness is regularly associated with septicaemia and involvement of the gut − the enteric fevers caused by S. *typhi* or S. *paratyphi* A, B and C.

S. *typhi* is the causative organism of typhoid fever, an essentially septicaemic illness lasting 3−5 weeks if untreated in which there are various focal manifestations. Infection is always acquired from a human source, usually urinary or faecal excretors. After ingestion the organisms penetrate the small intestinal mucosa and pass to the local lymph nodes. There the reticulo-endothelial macrophages mount a defence but if this is unsuccessful a persisting septicaemia commences, marking the termination of the incubation period (commonly 10−14 days). Initially symptoms are of fever (which may rise in a stepwise fashion), headache, impaired mentation, vague abdominal discomfort, constipation (not diarrhoea) and a nonproductive cough. Sometimes there may be no suggestive symptoms, the illness being initially a pyrexia of unknown origin. Later, after the seventh day of illness, crops of rose spots (caused by S. *typhi* emboli in the skin) may occur, as may splenomegaly. There may be seeding of organisms to form

metastatic foci in bones, in the bone marrow, in the lung and, most import-
antly, in the reticuloendothelial system: localization in the Peyer's patches
of the terminal ileum may cause haemorrhage or perforation or both.
S. typhi also localizes in the biliary tract and, especially in the presence of
gallstones, may cause persisting infection after the illness has resolved. This
can lead to continuous or intermittent excretion of the organisms in the bile
(and thus in the faeces) constituting an asymptomatic carrier state which
occurs in about 3–5% of typhoid fever patients.

Recognized complications of typhoid fever include femoral thrombophlebitis, cerebral thromboses, cholecystitis, pneumonia, osteomyelitis,
endocarditis and a 'toxic myocarditis' which may cause a bradycardia
relative to the fever.

Definitive diagnosis is made by culturing the organism from the blood.
Positive urine or stool culture may be found in chronic excretors ill with
other diseases. The Widal test may be suggestive, but both false positives
and false negatives may occur.

The treatment of first choice is usually chloramphenicol with co-
trimoxazole generally considered to be a very close second. Response to
therapy is usually slow, the fever and systemic symptoms taking 1–5 days
to resolve: even so haemorrhage and perforation at the site of Peyer's
patches may still occur despite continuing therapy. Classical signs of perforation may be minimal and a change from the characteristic typhoid
leukopenia to a leukocytosis is a helpful clue. Steroids may be used in
desperate situations to buy time and combat toxaemia.

Treatment of carriers tends to be disappointing: for faecal carriers (who
are not also urinary carriers) removal of a diseased gall bladder should be
advised, and if this fails a prolonged course of ampicillin or co-trimoxazole
may be tried. Even if apparently successful, permanent non-carriage
cannot be assumed as multiple stool cultures over a long period of time may
be negative only to be followed by transient or permanent excretion.

Paratyphoid tends to be a similar less severe illness with a lower incidence of serious complications. *Paratyphi B* may cause a florid crop of rose
spots.

Shigellae

There are four groups, *Shigella sonnei*, *S. flexneri*, *S. boydii* and *S. dysenteriae*. The first two are indigenous to Britain and all except *S. sonnei* are
more often than not imported infections. The shigellae are resistant to
gastric acid and relatively few organisms (e.g. 200 for *S. flexneri*) can initiate illnesses. The shigella organisms invade colonic epithelial cells, but
extra-colonic invasion does not usually occur.

The resulting illnesses are thus primarily colitic in nature with dysenteric
stools which may contain mucus, pus and blood. Vomiting is not usually a

prominent feature. In addition to the colitic component it has been postulated that an initial small bowel outpouring of fluid occurs because of an
adenyl cyclase mechanism somewhat similar to the cholera mechanism (see
Figure 11). Infection with S *dysenteriae* tends to be a more severe infection

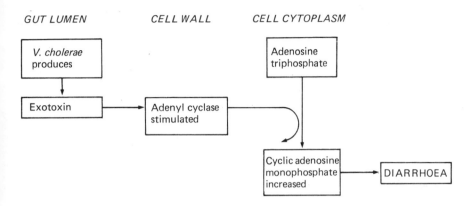

GUT LUMEN   CELL WALL   CELL CYTOPLASM

Figure 11   The biochemical pathogenesis of cholera. Cyclic adenosine monophosphate functions as a 'second messenger' and causes intestinal cells to secrete fluid
into the gut lumen

perhaps because it is the only strain known to produce a pathogenically
significant exotoxin.

Treatment depends on adequate fluid replacement and antibacterial
drugs probably should not be used routinely as most illnesses are self limiting and drug resistance rapidly occurs.

Pseudomonas

Most pseudomonas species are free living in nature. *Pseudomonas aeruginosa* is often found amongst the flora of the human gastrointestinal tract
and it is the pseudomonas species that most frequently becomes an oppor-
tunistic pathogen. *P. aeruginosa* infection constitutes the most problematical of nosocomial (hospital acquired) infections because:

(1)   It is resistant to (and may even grow in) commonly used disinfect-
ants.
(2)   It is resistant to commonly used antibacterial drugs.
(3)   The uninhibited use of the commonly used antibacterial drugs
allows it to flourish without competition from other bacteria.
(4)   It may be transmitted on medical and surgical equipment, and
(5)   Because it produces a large number of toxic extracellular products.

In man *P. aeruginosa* may colonize or invade the urinary tract, wounds, the skin (where it may produce haemorrhagic necrosis), burns, the lungs, the meninges and the bloodstream.

Treatment with antibacterial drugs is usually with the aminoglycosides (including gentamicin, tobramycin or amikacin) and also with carbenicillin or colistin. In future, immunization for at risk groups may well be practical — humoral immunity appears to be an important part of the host's defences.

Other pseudomonas organisms include *P. mallei* which causes glanders — a disease of horses which occasionally infects humans, and *P. pseudomallei* which produces a disease not unlike glanders.

Bordetella

There are two species of importance, *Bord. pertussis* (pertussis = intensive cough) and *Bord. parapertussis*. Bordetella grows exclusively in ciliated epithelial cells, thereby producing necrosis and tenacious mucus. As the organism is only isolated from about 50 % of patients in the whooping stage, it seems that the presence of the organism in large numbers is not required for perpetuation of the cough, and that other factors, such as toxin production, must be involved. There is little immunity gained from the mother by the transplacental route, and this lack is no doubt one contributing factor to the high mortality and morbidity in children under the age of six months.

Whooping cough, the illness produced by these organisms, is highly infectious, the attack rate among exposed non-immunized children being about 90 %. The incubation period is usually about 10–16 days.

The classical illness commences with a prodromal catarrhal stage lasting 7–14 days with sneezing, a mild cough and perhaps a slight fever. This stage then progresses to an afebrile paroxysmal 'whooping' stage which lasts for about 2 weeks. The whoops follows paroxysms of (expiratory) coughing which seemingly attempt to clear the airway of tenacious mucus which narrows and obstructs the lower respiratory tract. The child with 'near empty' lungs takes one or more large inspirations, which in passing through the narrowed airway, produces the classical whoop. The convalescent stage commonly lasts 2–3 weeks during which all symptoms and signs gradually resolve. Recurrence of whooping may subsequently occur with other (non-bordetella) respiratory tract infections.

Brucella

There are three main species: *Br. abortus*, *Br. mellitensis* and *Br. suis*. *Br. abortus* is the only species indigenous to Britain — the other two are occasionally imported in dairy products. British brucellosis is primarily an occupational disease which occurs in those in contact with cattle or dairy products. Either acute or chronic illness results in which the only common findings are of lymphadenopathy or splenomegaly which each occur in about 10% of patients.

Entry of the infection is via the gastrointestinal tract, skin, respiratory tract, conjunctivae or by accidental inoculation with live cattle vaccine. The organisms then pass to regional lymph nodes and into the blood, then localizing intracellularly in the liver, spleen, bone marrow, and lymphatic tissue where granuloma formation ensues. Symptoms are caused by release either of Brucella organisms or their antigens into the blood. Immune complex syndromes may also occur.

Culture of the organism from blood or tissue biopsy makes the diagnosis certain: however the organisms are notoriously difficult to grow and serological tests are useful, especially in the few patients who have no occupational exposure. Measurements of brucella specific immunoglobulins are now possible; if the brucella specific IgM level is raised the infection is probably active, and if the IgG level is raised this indicates that the patient has been infected at some stage. The major complications are psychiatric problems, debility, spondylitis, orchitis and endocarditis.

Treatment probably diminishes the severity and duration of acute episodes and may be helpful in chronic brucellosis. Therapies include streptomycin plus tetracycline in acute brucellosis and co-trimoxazole in both acute and chronic brucellosis. In chronic brucellosis tetracyclines are often used alone. Other antibacterial drugs await assessment, but hopefully the human disease will be eradicated by eliminating it in cattle.

Haemophilus

The major species associated with human disease is *H. influenzae* (Pfeiffer's bacillus). Contrary to the name *H. influenzae* does *not* cause influenza. The common illnesses produced include pharyngitis and laryngotracheitis in children and exacerbations of chronic bronchitis in adults.

Epiglottitis is usually caused by *H. influenzae* and can cause rapid respiratory obstruction − look for an enlarged red epiglottis and a localized respiratory 'whistle' which, on careful listening, is nearer to the ear than that of croup. (If epiglottitis is probable have facilities available for instant endotracheal intubation *before* inspecting the throat.)

Primary *H. influenzae* pneumonia does occur, but secondary pneumonia is more common, occurring secondary to chronic bronchitis, influenza, pertussis, measles and other virus infections with a respiratory component.

H. influenzae is a frequent cause of otitis media in children, especially the under fives, but is an uncommon cause in adults. Meningitis is also commonly caused by *H. influenzae* in young children: it is usually of slower onset than pneumococcal or meningococcal meningitis.

Other organisms include *H. aegyptius* which may cause a purulent conjunctivitis, *H. parainfluenzae*, a relatively minor pathogen which occasionally causes endocarditis, and *H. ducreyi* which causes chancroid, a venereal disease with localized 'soft sore' and regional lymphadenopathy.

Most strains of *H. influenzae* are susceptible to ampicillin but in rapidly mortal diseases such as meningitis even the low incidence of resistant strains becomes worrying and chloramphenicol is preferable as a first line therapy. Tetracyclines (which should not be given to young children) are usually effective especially in respiratory tract infection.

Yersinia (formerly Pasturella)

Y. pestis causes plague, an epidemic disease which is transmitted to humans from rodents by fleas. In the past widespread epidemics occurred with an associated high mortality. After being introduced by flea bite the bacilli pass to lymph nodes causing enlargement (*Bubonic* plague). Bloodstream spread occurs and with pulmonary involvement (*secondary pneumonic* plague) large numbers of bacilli are then coughed into the environment directly infecting the lungs of other humans to cause a *primary pneumonic* plague.

Control of disease demands suppression of rat populations and repeated vaccination of those at risk. Early antibacterial therapy is mandatory (within 12–15 hours of onset) as 'toxic' death may occur even after bacteriological cure. Drugs utilized include tetracyclines, streptomycin and chloramphenicol.

Yersinia pseudotuberculosis may produce a mesenteric adenitis which mimics appendicitis or may cause a bacteraemic illness.

Y. enterocolitica resembles *Y. pseudotuberculosis* and may cause terminal ileitis, mesenteric adenitis, appendicitis, erythema nodosum and either mild or severe diarrhoeal illnesses.

Y. multocida is pathogenic for a wide range of animals. Human infection occasionally results secondary to dog or cat bites: the infected wounds are painful and suppurate, and may later become necrotic. Bloodstream spread may occur resulting in metastatic focal lesions. Penicillin is usually curative.

Vibrios

Vibrio cholerae is a strict parasite of man which causes asymptomatic infection or clinical cholera. Several strains exist including Inaba and Ogawa serotypes of both the classical and El Tor biotypes. *V. cholerae* produces a variety of extracellular products and causes a purely biochemical (exotoxin) induced diarrhoea (Figure 11). There is no tissue invasion. Spread occurs by water or less commonly by food which is contaminated with human excreta. The incubation period varies from a few hours to a few days and the hallmark of severe cholera is a copious watery diarrhoea with flakes of thick mucus therein, giving rise to 'rice water' stools. Rapid and devastating loss of fluid and electrolytes occurs with hypovolaemic shock and acidosis.

Treatment is by replacement of lost fluid and electrolytes. Tetracyclines effectively clear the gut of organisms. Vaccines confer short duration type-specific immunity.

V. parahaemolyticus causes a vomiting and diarrhoeal illness and is usually associated with seafood products.

Treponemataceae

There are three main genera: Treponema, Borrelia and Leptospira.

Treponema pallidum is the only treponemal infection indigenous to Britain: it causes syphilis. The basic tissue reaction to this organism is infiltration with lymphocytes, plasma cells and macrophages with proliferation of fibroblasts.

Congenital syphilis is caused by transplacental infection and may be manifest at birth by wasting, rashes, epiphysitis, pneumonia, liver fibrosis, meningovascular problems and cerebral dysfunction. In later childhood periostitis and iridocyclitis can occur and often there may be later development of tooth deformities (Hutchinson's peg incisors, Moon's domed molars), interstitial keratitis, nerve dysfunction (deafness or blindness), gumma formation, general paralysis of the insane, or tabes dorsalis.

Genitally acquired syphilis (the Great Pox) is acquired when *T. pallidum* enters the body via minute epithelial abrasions or by penetrating intact mucous membranes or possibly via unbroken skin. It can be divided into three stages.

(1) In primary syphilis a primary chancre may be noted 10–90 days after infection. Classically a chancre is a single superficial painless ulcer, which does not bleed spontaneously, is indurated and which heals quickly with minimal scarring. Numerous treponemes are present and regional lymphadenopathy is painless and rubbery. The *T. pallidum* are disseminated throughout the body at the stage of the primary chancre.

(2) In about a third of patients with primary syphilis, secondary syphilis will occur, usually 1–3 months later. Symptoms and signs, if they occur, are usually transient and include pyrexia, malaise, lymphadenopathy, alopecia, snail track ulcers, retinitis, iritis, iridocyclitis, warts (condylomata lata) and a maculopapular rash which is classically bilateral, copper coloured and non-itchy.

(3) Tertiary syphilis may occur 3–25 years later. Few treponemes are present as tissue destruction is largely on an immune basis, with gumma formation and interstitial inflammation. Gummas are localized firm rubbery masses when situated in solid tissues, but if present on body surfaces they manifest as indolent punched out ulcers with a 'wash leather' base. Interstitial inflammation leads to chronic degeneration and atrophy in the nervous system. *Meningovascular syphilis* is associated with an endarteritis obliterans whereas *parenchymatous syphilis* damages central nervous system tissue and causes general paralysis of the insane or tabes dorsalis. *Cardiovascular syphilis* usually manifests as aortitis – a medial necrosis secondary to endarteritis obliterans of the vasa vasorum.

Diagnosis in primary and secondary syphilis can be made by seeing the organism on dark ground illumination or by using immunofluorescent techniques. Numerous serological tests are available and the reader is advised to consult specialist texts for detailed information. Essentially two tests are generally used, one which becomes positive early after infection and which usually becomes negative after treatment (such as the Venereal Disease Reference Laboratory test – VDRL), combined with a specific test with no biological false positives which becomes positive later in the course of illness and which tends to persist, thus providing a marker of infection whether past or present (for example the *Treponema pallidum* Haemagglutination test – TPHA).

Treatment is usually with penicillin: in the penicillin allergic patient tetracyclines are useful but are contraindicated in children and pregnant females, for whom erythromycin is a suitable alternative. Reactions to treatment sometimes occur in established syphilis (Jarisch–Herxheimer reactions) and steroids may need to be given to avoid exacerbation of symptoms and signs which may occur in this reaction.

Borrelia

There are several species of this organism and each produces a relapsing fever in which there are recurrent febrile paroxysms with intervals of apparent recovery.

Leptospira

Ingestion of, or direct exposure to, urine of infected animals may cause illness which is usually of abrupt onset. In severe forms the capillary epithelium becomes swollen and has increased permeability which leads to oedema, hypoxia and haemorrhages. Many systems can be involved: jaundice may result from a combination of cholestasis, haemolysis and liver damage, kidney tubule damage may cause oliguria, meningeal involvement may cause headache and meningism, and muscle involvement may cause myocarditis. Haemorrhage can occur from various sites to produce epistaxis, ecchymoses, petechiae, haematemesis, melaena or conjunctival haemorrhages. When a severe multisystem illness with jaundice results the eponym Weil's disease is applied.

The causative organism of leptospirosis is *Leptospira interrogans* and in Britain three main species are responsible for clinical illness. *L. hebdomadis*, *L. canicola* (which typically causes abrupt onset of fever possibly with meningism) and *L. icterohaemorrhagica* (which is commonly acquired from rat's urine). The latter organism may cause three main syndromes, an abrupt onset febrile illness, jaundice with or without renal failure, or a meningitis illness: combinations often occur.

Diagnosis is by dark ground illumination, serology, or by culture of the organism involved. *L. hebdomadis* is hardly ever cultured and the diagnosis is confirmed serologically.

Treatment is with penicillin or tetracyclines, but bacteriological cure may not cure the illness. If renal impairment is severe temporary dialysis may be required.

OTHER NOTABLE PATHOGENIC BACTERIA

Actinomyces

In common with nocardia these organisms were thought to be fungi (eumycetes) but they are now recognized to be bacteria and are thus called pseudomycetes. *Actinomyces israelii*, an anaerobic organism, causes actinomycosis which occasionally causes 'lumpy jaws' with pus resembling sulphur granules. Thoracic and abdominal disease may also occur with pus draining from multiple sinuses. Treatment is with long term penicillin combined with suitable drainage. Tetracycline or erythromycin are also useful.

Campylobacter

These organisms cause a diarrhoeal illness often with a febrile prodromal period and frequently with severe abdominal pain. Infection often appears to be from animal sources, particularly poultry.

Francisella (Pasteurella) tularensis

This organism produces tularaemia, a highly infectious illness usually resulting from the handling of infected animals. Characteristically a necrotic skin or mucous membrane lesion develops at the inoculation site and there is regional lymph node enlargement, septicaemia and marked fever. Treatment is usually with streptomycin.

Legionnaires' disease

Legionnaires' disease is a recently recognized bacterial pneumonia which appears to occur sporadically and in outbreaks. It has a predilection for elderly males, especially those who smoke. Systemic symptoms may be prominent with severe malaise, myalgia, abdominal or chest pain and headache. Clouding of consciousness without respiratory failure is suggestive. Chest signs are variable and chest X-ray often shows patchy infiltrations possibly with effusions. The white cell count is usually raised and other suggestive features include gastrointestinal symptoms, an ESR in excess of 80 mm per hour, proteinuria, hyponatraemia and a raised blood urea. Serological tests confirm the diagnosis. Early suspicion is important as the treatment of choice appears to be erythromycin which is not a usual first-line choice for 'typical' bacterial pneumonias.

Mixed infections

A double infection with *Fusobacterium fusiforme* and *Borrelia vincentii* may cause Vincent's angina, an ulcerative gingivostomatitis which often occurs opportunistically.

Treatment is with penicillin or metronidazole in association with oral hygiene, including mouth washes.

Mycoplasma

These organisms are *not* true bacteria but appear to resemble bacteria which permanently lack a cell wall: they are thus resistant to antibacterial agents that attack cell walls. The most common serious disease produced is 'atypical' (Eaton agent) pneumonia with fever, cough, mucoid sputum and X-ray changes which are typically more extensive than clinical examination would have suggested.

Treatment is with tetracyclines or erythromycin.

Nocardia

Unlike actinomyces these are aerobic. Abscess formation is usual, often occurring in the lung, and producing an illness resembling pulmonary tuberculosis or actinomycosis.

COMMONLY USED ANTIBACTERIAL DRUGS: A BRIEF REVIEW

The following account does *not* attempt to provide a comprehensive account of the characteristics, uses and dosages of antibacterial drugs: for these the reader is referred to more specialized texts.

Successful drug use against any human parasite depends on two factors. *Selective toxicity* – the drug must be *available at the site of infection* at *an effective concentration*. To be effective the appropriate antibacterial drug must be administered in an adequate dosage at correct intervals for a sufficient period of time.

The aminoglycosides

All of this class of drug act on protein synthetic mechanisms. Those administered parenterally accumulate if there is renal failure and may cause ear damage.

Amikacin. The major use seems to be for gentamicin resistant gram-negative infections.

Gentamicin. This drug has to be given parenterally, usually for severe infections with gram-negative bacilli, particularly *Pseudomonas aeruginosa* infections. It is especially useful for 'informed guess' initial treatment of infections likely to be caused by gram-negative bacilli, or in septicaemic states before the organism responsible has been identified – in which case combination therapy is often required (usually with a penicillin and/or metronidazole). Other uses include urinary tract infections (the urine should be alkaline for best effect), staphylococcal infections and in combinations for bacterial endocarditis. It is not reliably effective against streptococcal infections.

Neomycin has been used for bowel 'sterilization', topical treatment of skin infections and intestinal infections. For each of these uses there are theoretical and practical disadvantages.

Streptomycin has its main use in the treatment of tuberculosis. It is also used against plague, tularaemia and in combinations against brucella infection.

Tobramycin has a possibly greater intrinsic activity than gentamicin against *Pseudomonas aeruginosa*.

The cephalosporins

Like penicillins these inhibit bacterial cell wall synthesis and are thus bactericidal.

They are useful alternatives to penicillin. Common uses include staphylococcal infections including those caused by penicillinase producing bacteria, streptococcal infections, urinary tract infections, gonorrhoea, syphilis, and in gram-negative septicaemias providing the sensitivities of the causative organism(s) are known.

Derivatives of cephalosporins and of the related cephamycins abound. Cefoxitin seems likely to be a very useful drug as its spectrum of activity includes anaerobic organisms (including *Bacteroides fragilis*).

Chloramphenicol

Chloramphenicol is a potent inhibitor of bacterial protein synthesis.

It has an extremely broad spectrum including anaerobic organisms such as *Bacteroides fragilis*. *Pseudomonas aeruginosa* is notably resistant. It is a useful drug for severe infections when the small risk of precipitating aplastic anaemia is relatively less important. Its common uses include typhoid fever (for which it is widely regarded as the treatment of choice), other salmonella infections in which chemotherapy is indicated, rickettsial diseases, some klebsiella infections, melioidosis and eye infections. There are very few indications for non-topical use of this drug in General Practice. In *Haemophilus influenzae* meningitis chloramphenicol is more reliable than high dose ampicillin. It is also useful in pyogenic meningitis if for any reason the causative organism cannot be rapidly identified.

Clindamycin and lincomycin

These are usually used to treat staphylococcal and bacteroides infections. The risk of precipitating pseudomembranous colitis has caused many to choose alternative therapies.

Co-trimoxazole

This is a combination of trimethoprim and sulphamethoxazole in a ratio of 1:5. Each constituent is bacteriostatic, acting at different levels of bacterial folic acid synthesis, and in combination the effect is often bactericidal.

Common clinical uses include urinary tract infections (particularly as the potentially reinfecting bowel flora have little chance of developing resistance to two drugs simultaneously), lower respiratory tract infections, typhoid, brucellosis, gonorrhoea, toxoplasmosis (a protozoa), plague and nocardia infections.

Erythromycin

This drug interferes with bacterial protein synthesis at the ribosome level.

Common clinical uses include streptococcal and pneumococcal infections in penicillin allergic patients, otitis media, some staphylococcal infections, mycoplasma pneumonia and elimination of diphtheria in carriers. It, like co-trimoxazole, *may* possibly attenuate whooping cough if given early enough in the illness: it *may* also reduce infectivity of established cases and its use prophylactically for close contacts is in theory likely to be effective.

Fusidic acid

Fusidic acid is an inhibitor of bacterial protein synthesis.

It is only used in staphylococcal infections, when it is perhaps best used in combination to avoid emergence of fucidin-resistant strains.

Methenamine mandelate and hippurate

These exert their main effect by liberation of formaldehyde (to which all microorganisms are vulnerable) in the urinary tract.

The only use is in urinary tract infections − the urine must be acidified for maximum effect.

Metronidazole

Metronidazole is active against anaerobic bacteria, including *Bacteroides fragilis* and anaerobic streptococci. It is inactive against aerobic and facultatively anaerobic bacteria.

Its main clinical usage is in anaerobic sepsis particularly if this has a large bowel origin. As it is relatively non-toxic it is often used in broad spectrum antibiotic 'cocktails'. It is also used in Vincent's angina.

Nitrofurantoin

This drug is rapidly excreted in the urine and its only clinical use is in urinary tract infections, particularly those caused by *E. coli*.

Penicillins

These valuable drugs block bacterial cell wall synthesis and thus only attack actively growing bacteria.

Common clinical uses include *Strep. pyogenes* infections (which are almost invariably sensitive), *Strep. pneumoniae* infections including otitis media in older children and adults, some bacterial meningitises (penicillin can be used alone in proven meningococcal and pneumococcal meningitis), some puerperal infections, bacterial endocarditis caused by sensitive organisms, *Clostridium perfringens* and *tetani* infections, anthrax, gonorrhoea, syphilis, actinomycosis and leptospirosis. Penicillin can be used as prophylaxis against bacterial endocarditis and rheumatic fever.

Certain organisms, particularly 'hospital' staphylococci, are penicillin G resistant as they produce penicillinase, and drugs which are unaffected by penicillinase (e.g. flucloxacillin, methicillin or non-penicillin drugs) have to be used.

Ampicillin and ampicillin-like compounds (such as amoxycillin and talampicillin) have a broader antibacterial spectrum than penicillin alone, including infections caused by many gram-negative bacilli, particularly some strains of *E. coli*. Common uses include urinary tract infections, lower respiratory tract infections (especially as 'informed guess' therapy in exacerbations of chronic bronchitis), biliary tract infections, otitis media in young children in whom *H. influenzae* is a common pathogen, attempted eradication of the typhoid carrier state, gram-negative septicaemias, bacterial endocarditis, gonorrhoea and against *Listeria monocytogenes*.

Carbenicillin is usually used in combination treatments of pseudomonas infections: there are several other recently introduced extended-spectrum penicillins which are active against pseudomonas.

Rifampicin

Rifampicin acts by inhibiting bacterial RNA synthesis.

Common uses include the treatment of tuberculosis, leprosy and meningococcal carrier states. It is also active against trachoma (a chlamydia) and *in vitro* against certain viruses. In Britain its major use is confined to therapy of tuberculosis.

Sulphonamides

Sulphonamides are bacteriostatic and act by competitive inhibition of folate synthesis by bacterial cells. This action is selectively toxic to the bacteria as their cells appear to be impermeable to folic acid, whereas mammalian cells can utilize preformed dietary folic acid. Sulphonamides can also be used against some protozoal organisms.

The only common use of sulphonamides as a single therapy is in urinary tract infections. Sulphonamides can be used prophylactically for rheumatic fever and for meningococcal meningitis if the current strains of meningococci are known to be sulphonamide sensitive.

Tetracyclines

These are bacteriostatic, inhibiting bacterial protein synthesis on the ribosomes.

Tetracyclines stain the teeth of children and therefore should not be given to them *or* to pregnant women.

Common uses include lower respiratory tract infections, gonorrhoea and non-specific urethritis, brucellosis, biliary tract infections, mycoplasma pneumonia, eradication of *Vibrio cholerae*, rickettsial infections, Q fever and psittacosis. Other possible uses are in the treatment of relapsing fever, melioidosis, actinomycosis, *Cl. perfringens* infections, anthrax, lepto-spirosis, tropical sprue and acne vulgaris.

Suggested further reading

Smith, H. (1977). *Antibiotics in Clinical Practice.* (Tunbridge Wells: Pitman Medical Publishing Co.)

Cruicshank, R., Duguid, J.P., Marmion, R.H. and Swain, R.H.A. (1973). *Medical Microbiology.* (Edinburgh: Churchill Livingstone)

3
Viral infections

Viral infections may cause acute illness, chronic illness, some degenerative diseases, some neoplasms and may initiate or contribute towards some immune responses.

The word virus is derived from a Latin word meaning poison, an appropriate derivation as virus particles *outside* living cells exhibit no characteristics of living organisms and function only as complex chemicals. They differ from conventional poisons in that once *inside* a living cell they synthesize rather than destroy by interfering with the host cell's synthetic mechanisms (Figures 12(a) and 12(b)). The basic structure of an archetypal extracellular virus is shown in Figure 13.

The external coat protects the virus and enables it to attach and penetrate potential host cells: such penetration may only occur in certain types of host cells but some viruses (Lassa fever virus for example) are pantropic and may penetrate and damage most if not all of the host tissues. After entry into a host cell the virus uncoats and the contents are released.

The capsid is a protein containing layer which encloses the viral nucleic acid: it is composed of capsomeres (identical building blocks) which are usually assembled in a regular fashion − thus causing most viruses to have a degree of symmetry.

49

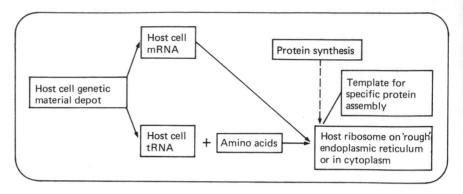

Figure 12(a)   The normal host cell mechanism of protein synthesis (Adapted from *Update*, with permission)

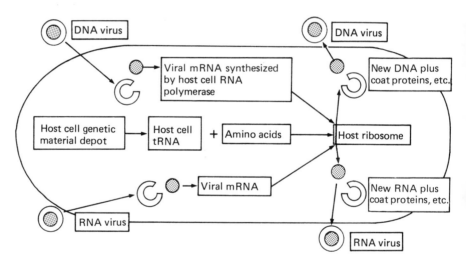

Figure 12(b)   A simplified account of virus-induced host cell protein synthesis

The core consists of either deoxyribonucleic acid (DNA) or ribonucleic acid (RNA): upon liberation the DNA or RNA utilizes the host cell's synthetic machinery and cellular substrates to produce various substances including those required for viral replication. Both DNA and RNA viruses ultimately intervene at the level of messenger RNA by insertion of their foreign genetic information (Figure 12(b)).

Each part of the virus may be antigenic and elicit host antibody responses which may be important in the development of host immunity. In addition the viral invasion may alter the host cell surface antigens by the presence of residual viral antigens or modification of the host's antigens.

Core
(DNA or RNA
— not both)

Capsid (the protein coat of
the core) consisting of
"building blocks" called   capsomeres

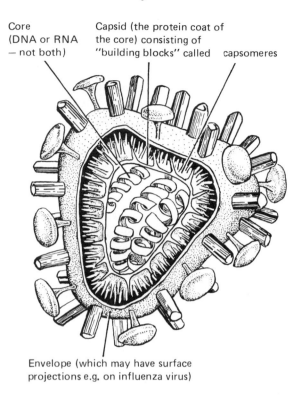

Envelope (which may have surface
projections e.g. on influenza virus)

Figure 13   Schematic diagram of a mature virus particle (virion) (Adapted from *Update*, with permission)

MECHANISMS OF VIRAL PATHOGENICITY

(1)   *Direct attack by the host on cells containing the virus.* Virus induced antigens present on the host cell may be recognized as foreign by the host. An immune response may then be mounted against the foreign antigens with destruction of the cell bearing these antigens.

(2)   *Activation of trigger mechanisms* can result in inflammation, hypersensitivity reactions and (in the case of complement activation) host cell destruction.

(3)   *Virus-antibody complex formation*, perhaps involving complement, may cause problems if the complexes are deposited in tissues or organs. Many viruses have been implicated in immune complex formation.

(4)   *The host's immunological responses may be altered*, especially by viral infections which attack lymphocytes, thereby affecting either cell mediated immunity or antibody production or both. Tempor-

51

ary immunosuppression may result (as in measles), immune mediated diseases may be initiated, as may some 'chronic degenerative' diseases.

(5) *The host cell's nucleic acid may be disrupted*: if such disruption is mild either chronic cellular instability results or immune mediated diseases may occur. If disruption is severe cell death may result. Malignant neoplasia, one of the as yet unsolved problems of mankind, may at least in part have viral infection as a necessary, if not as a causative, requirement. There is strong evidence that Burkitt's lymphoma and nasopharyngeal carcinoma have Epstein–Barr virus infection as one precipitating factor. Cervical carcinoma has an association with human Herpes virus type 2 infection.

Certain viruses produce slowly progressive illnesses perhaps by chronic interference and 'pseudointegration' with host cell chromosomes or by chronic aggravation of the infected cells. Table 2 details some diseases possibly associated with such 'slow virus' infections. A slow virus aetiology has been speculated for motor neurone disease and indeed poliovirus-like particles have been identified in anterior horn cells of the spinal cord.

Table 2 Some diseases possibly associated with slow virus infections

Creutzfeldt–Jakob disease	Transmissible agent demonstrated
Kuru	Transmissible agent demonstrated
Systemic lupus erythematosus	Paramyxoviruses associated*
Multiple sclerosis	Measles virus associated
Progressive multifocal leucoencephalopathy	SV 40 type virus associated
Subacute sclerosing panencephalitis	Measles virus associated

*Associated is not synonymous with 'caused by'.

The host's principal defences against virus and other infections have been outlined previously (Chapter 1) but recovery from some viral infections occurs too rapidly for reactive antibody to be implicated. Once antibody to a specific strain of a particular virus has been formed immunity to reinfection and clinical illness is usually, but not always, of long duration.

Laboratory confirmation of infection with a particular virus is usually more expeditiously performed by serological tests: isolation and typing of viruses is in general more tedious and in certain instances involves risk as laboratory exposure to the virus itself (rather than its antibody) is involved. However virus isolation and typing are necessary when new epidemic strains arise (as serological tests often do not differentiate between closely related viruses). Microscopic observation of different effects on various cell cultures (including embryonic kidney, lung fibroblast and HeLa cell lines) may give a provisional identification of the virus concerned.

A CLINICALLY BIASED ACCOUNT OF COMMON PATHOGENIC VIRUSES

Figure 14 is a classification of most viruses pathogenic to humans. Differentiation is made between DNA and RNA viruses: at the present stage of antiviral chemotherapy such a differentiation (unlike Gram's bacterial staining) is not useful either diagnostically or (with certain exceptions) therapeutically, but in future such differentiation may become relevant.

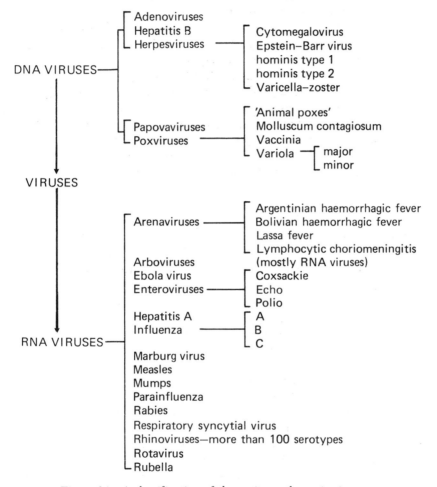

Figure 14   A classification of the major pathogenic viruses

Adenovirus infections

Adenoviruses, of which there are more than 30 serotypes pathogenic for man, were first isolated from adenoidal tissue − hence the name. They have affinity for lymphoid tissue, the respiratory tract, the gastrointestinal tract and the conjunctivae. Most infections are of acute onset, self limiting and are rarely fatal. Illnesses produced by adenoviruses rarely provide clinically diagnostic features, but there are several patterns of disease that may occur.

Acute feverish respiratory diseases of children have an incubation period of 2–5 days and may present with fever alone, pharyngitis, tracheitis, bronchitis or pneumonia. These adenovirus infections are probably the most common cause of non-diagnosable childhood fevers. Adenovirus infection is thought to cause 2–7% of respiratory tract infections in young children.

Acute respiratory disease, a disease which tends to occur in mini-epidemics, consists of fever, pharyngitis with or without lymph node enlargement, and pneumonia. The usual incubation period is 5–6 days and the illness lasts for up to 10 days.

Epidemic keratoconjunctivitis is usually caused by adenovirus Type 8 which causes ocular folliculitis, eyelid oedema, photophobia and lachrymation.

Pharyngoconjunctival fever is usually caused by Type 3 or 7 adenovirus which infects the eyes and the tonsils – possibly causing tonsillar exudates with regional lymph node enlargement.

Other illnesses associated with adenovirus infections include acute haemorrhagic cystitis and intussusception in children.

In view of the large numbers of adenoviruses, antibody testing for specific strains is impractical as a screening procedure, but fortunately all adenovirus strains share cross-reacting complement fixing antigens: such antigens cause only a brief response in complement fixation tests and thus positive titres are strong evidence of acute infection. Other tests available include neutralization and haemagglutination inhibition tests which are type specific and tend to remain positive for longer. In practice isolation and typing of the virus concerned are a necessary preliminary before screening paired sera for rising titres using serotype specific neutralization or haemagglutination inhibition tests which relate a specific adenovirus serotype to a particular illness. Demonstration of rising antibody titres is essential because, after an acute infection, the adenovirus is often shed for prolonged periods (particularly from the gastrointestinal tract) and thus isolation of virus is not necessarily of diagnostic significance during an illness.

Some adenoviruses are oncogenic (i.e. cause neoplasia) in laboratory animals.

Hepatitis B ('Serum hepatitis')

This is a disease classically transmitted by blood or blood products, infected needles (drug addicts and the tattooed) and by sexual contact. The virus is present in many bodily secretions and transmission may occur by continued 'household exposure' to carriers of the Hepatitis B virus. Hepatitis B is a hazard for hospital staff, particularly those in close contact with patients or products related to patients whose immune systems are abnormal.

The incubation period is about 40–180 days, longer than that of hepatitis A. Clinically there is a prodromal illness of up to 2 weeks consisting of nausea, malaise, anorexia and fever. Transient arthralgia and skin rashes may occur (as in hepatitis A) which are thought to be related to immune complex deposition. Two major factors influence the severity of the illness produced: younger patients usually have a milder illness, and large infecting doses of virus usually cause more severe illness.

The pathogenesis of hepatitis B is multifactorial but it appears that hepatic necrosis is mediated by T lymphocytes reacting with the hepatitis B virus surface antigen on the surface of infected cells. There are at least three antigens relevant to hepatitis B virus infection.

(1) Hepatitis B surface antigen (HBs Ag) which is the commonly used marker of hepatitis B virus infection. In general the HBs Ag is present in the blood 1–7 weeks (average 4-weeks) before and 1–6 weeks after the onset of acute hepatitis. Antibody to the antigen (anti HBs) appears during convalescence from hepatitis B.
(2) Hepatitis B core antigen (HBc Ag).
(3) 'Little' e antigen (HBe Ag). This is a valuable marker of infectivity.

Acute hepatitis B often presents as a classical hepatitis with jaundice, but other patterns of illness may result:

(1) The hepatitis may be anticteric and thus unlikely to be diagnosed unless liver function tests are performed. Many patients who are discovered to be HBs Ag carriers cannot recall an attack of hepatitis.
(2) A predominantly cholestatic picture may result.
(3) The hepatitis may relapse: this usually occurs within 3 months of recovery from the initial infection.
(4) A fulminant hepatitis of high mortality may supervene: this is often associated with a brisk immunological response to the virus – which indeed may have been cleared from the blood prior to presentation.
(5) Subacute hepatic necrosis may develop: this may resolve or progress inexorably.
(6) Chronic persistent hepatitis may follow: this is usually benign and self limiting.
(7) The patient may make an apparent complete recovery but continue to carry the virus: permanent carriage is likely if the HBs Ag is not eliminated within 13 weeks after an acute hepatitis.

Herpesvirus infections

There are four herpesvirus infections common in man: Cytomegalovirus (CMV), Epstein-Barr virus (EBV), Herpes simplex virus (HSV) and Varicella–zoster virus (VZV). All four have the ability to persist in hosts after an acute infection with possible chronic infection or reactivation.

A fifth infection, *Herpesvirus simiae*, an infection of monkeys, may occasionally cause a high mortality encephalitis in humans.

Cytomegalovirus infections

The name derives from the finding of large cells with intranuclear inclusion bodies found in various infected tissues. Most infections are asymptomatic (or undiagnosed) and occur in childhood. Sixty to 90% of adults have experienced CMV infection. Prolonged excretion of the virus may occur despite high serum antibody levels.

Primary infection of the mother during pregnancy *may* result in congenital infection which *may* result in subsequent clinical illness of the child. Classical signs of intrauterine infection include low birth weight, hepatomegaly, splenomegaly, microcephaly, mental retardation, motor disability, jaundice, petechiae, choroidoretinitis and periventricular cerebral calcification.

In 'fit' adults a heterophil antibody negative infectious mononucleosis syndrome may occur with lymph node enlargement and atypical lymphocytes in the blood. Associated pharyngitis is uncommon. Hepatitis (in which fever and jaundice may coexist) may result, as may encephalitis, pneumonitis, erythema multiforme or the Guillain–Barré syndrome.

Infection in the immunosuppressed, particularly in renal transplant patients, and in those who have received blood transfusions, may cause 2–3 weeks of 'fever of uncertain origin', hepatitis, hepatosplenomegaly, lymph node enlargement or a pneumonitis (which may be confused with pneumocystis carinii in the immunosuppressed). Bizarre immunological reactions occur which confuse the serologically orientated diagnostician.

Isolation of the virus, although suggestive, does not necessarily imply a recent infection as excretion of the virus, particularly in the urine, may be chronic. Serological tests (particularly a raised IgM) or significant changes in paired sera antibody levels are necessary for confirmation of active infection.

There is no specific treatment.

Epstein–Barr virus infection (Infectious mononucleosis)

Infections acquired in early childhood tend to be mild and are often unrecognized, whereas infections in older age groups tend to be more severe. The incubation period is 30–50 days and after a brief period of non-specific malaise there follows fever (which may last for 7–10 days and occasionally longer), tender lymph node enlargement, splenomegaly in about 50% of cases, pharyngitis, tonsillitis with a white exudate confined to the tonsillar area, commonly palatal petechiae, a blood picture of mononucleosis (50% or more of lymphocytes with at least 10 per cent of atypical forms and perhaps an elevation of the total white cell count), and the production of heterophil antibodies. The Paul–Bunnell test reveals the presence of these antibodies (which may only be evident late in the course of illness) which agglutinate sheep erythrocytes, are absorbed by ox erythrocytes but not by guinea pig kidney cells. About 70% of patients have a positive heterophil antibody test during the first three weeks of illness. The Paul–Bunnell test has been largely superceded by a more simple variation – the monospot test.

Hepatomegaly occurs in about 10% of patients, and disorders of liver function tests are common but jaundice only occurs in about 5% of patients. Occasionally isolated fever, lymph node enlargement, or pharyngitis may each be the only evidence of infection.

Kissing, perhaps with an exchange of cells containing the virus, appears to be a major mode of transmission. After infection the virus persists in the throat but there is only a low yield of extracellular virus – thus the duration of infectivity after an attack is unpredictable.

It is thought that the clinical manifestations are caused by T lymphocyte reactions to B lymphocytes whose cell membranes have been altered by EBV infection – the atypical lymphocytes are both B and T cells. Associated with EBV infection there is a temporary depression of cell mediated immunity and there is also a notable *temporary* hypersensitivity to ampicillin and its derivatives which causes a skin rash in the majority of patients to whom this drug has been given. An erythematous maculopapular rash, often seen on the trunk and proximal limbs, may occur in the early stages of EBV infection (without exposure to ampicillin).

Complications include airway obstruction, splenic rupture, thrombocytopenia, pneumonitis, myocarditis, nephritis and the Guillain–Barré syndrome which may lead to respiratory paralysis. A meningo-encephalitis may occur. Chronic 'complications' in certain specific circumstances include Burkitt's lymphoma and nasopharyngeal carcinoma.

For practical purposes a positive Paul–Bunnell or monospot test is confirmatory of EBV infection: false positives do occur but are rare. If diagnostic doubt persists specific EBV antibody studies can be performed – a raised IgM, which disappears within a few weeks, is suggestive of recent infection. If all EBV studies are negative cytomegalovirus infection or toxoplasmosis are diagnostic possibilities as both can produce similar syndromes. Therapy is symptomatic. Complications require treatment in their own right: impending respiratory obstruction can be treated with steroids or, if obstruction is imminent, with nasolaryngo/tracheal intubation.

Steroids, although undoubtedly effective, should probably not be used to treat the profound malaise that can be associated with EBV infection, especially as the long-term implications of such immunointerference are unknown.

Herpes simplex virus infections

There are two herpes simplex viruses, both of which have an average incubation period of six days (range 2–20). In general HSV type 1 causes infections above the waist, whilst HSV type 2 causes infections below the waist: both can occur in the presence of significant serum antibody levels. When infection is confined to the skin there are small thin-walled vesicles containing clear fluid which may be on an erythematous base, but if such lesions occur in mucous membranes they tend to break down to form erosions or ulcers. Scar formation is unusual in the absence of secondary infection. Both types of virus may cause meningitis, encephalitis, radiculitis, myelitis or eye infections with a possibly recurrent keratitis with dendritic ulcers and conjunctivitis. Disseminated infection may occur in neonates, whereas patients with eczema may have widespread skin infection (eczema herpeticum or Kaposi's varicelliform eruption).

Herpes simplex virus probably does not survive for long outside the body except in skin scabs shed from eczema herpeticum which may harbour the intact virus for a brief period.

Diagnosis is usually clinical, but may be confirmed by isolation and identification of the virus or by finding significant titre changes in serological tests.

Topical treatment is with idoxuridine in dimethylsulphoxide or with intravenous adenine arabinoside if generalized spread of infection has occurred.

HSV type 1 infection is common. Primary infections mostly pass unnoticed but (usually in children) a painful gingivostomatitis may result, classically with fever, serpiginous ulcers in the front and back of the mouth and with associated cervical gland enlargement. Recurrent herpes labialis (cold sores) are the commonest manifestation of HSV infection and they often occur in association with physical irritation, fevers, menstruation or stress. Recurrent intra-oral HSV infections are rare, such lesions being more commonly due to 'idiopathic' aphthous ulceration.

Traumatic injection of virus into the skin can give rise to painful lesions of the fingers – herpetic whitlows: dentists, anaesthetists and nurses are at particular occupational risk as they are often exposed to HSV in the mouths of patients.

HSV type 2 is usually transmitted venereally or acquired by perinates from the maternal birth canal – caesarian section should be considered if active maternal infection is present.

In the female, infection is usually of the cervix with possible vulval and vaginal involvement. Symptoms tend to be recurrent and include fever, dysuria, leukorrhoea, soreness and inguinal node enlargement: infection confined to the cervix is commonly asymptomatic. There is an association between HSV type 2 and cervical carcinoma. In the male vesicles and ulcers may occur on the glans, prepuce and shaft of the penis. In both sexes lesions of HSV type 2 may occur elsewhere on the body depending on varied sexual practices.

There is no cure for genital herpes: the use of 5-idoxuridine has been disappointing.

Varicella-zoster virus infection

This virus causes chickenpox, or herpes zoster (shingles). Both these VZV infections are moderately infectious in that they each may result in chickenpox in contacts. Shingles, in theory at least, cannot be transmitted from person to person.

Chickenpox is a common childhood illness — an occupational hazard of attending school. Infection is primarily by droplet spread from the respiratory tract but the early skin lesions are also infectious. After an incubation period ranging from 11 to 20 days a brief prodromal period may occur followed by 1–6 days of crops of superficial pruritic macules which rapidly evolve through papular and vesicular stages to form pustules. These later dry and crust. The rash classically starts on the face and scalp and spreads to the trunk: it is thus relatively centripetal (centre seeking), and tends to be more marked in eczematous areas and in other areas where skin irritation has occurred — particularly sunburn. Residual scarring is rare in the absence of secondary infection or scratching. Lesions may also occur in the respiratory tract, the oropharynx, the gastrointestinal tract and vagina.

The cropping possibly results from cyclical viraemia and in the prodromal period a fleeting erythematous rash may occur presumably representing a response to early viraemia.

Chickenpox is probably infectious for several days before the rash and is infectious until the last lesion has crusted.

Complications include pneumonia, thrombocytopenia, secondary bacterial infection and encephalitis which has a predilection for the cerebellum.

The clinical picture is often diagnostic but in questionable cases electron microscopy of vesicle fluid may be suggestive and serves to differentiate from smallpox. Rises in complement fixing antibody are diagnostic (as long as HSV titres are static). If such tests are not diagnostic the more specific neutralization tests can be used.

Prophylactic immunoglobulin shortly after exposure reduces the attack rate and modifies the severity of chickenpox. Transplacental transmission of maternal antibody gives neonates protection for about 6 months. Adenine arabinoside is indicated for extensive disease in patients with impaired immunity.

Herpes zoster is caused by reactivation of VZV initially acquired during a previous attack of chickenpox: the VZV is harboured in the dorsal sensory ganglia as a *persistent* infection (viruses continuously being elaborated) or by *latent* infection (no replication). After reactivation the virus travels down the sensory nerves thereby causing prodromal pain and paraesthesia of dermatome distribution. Upon arrival in the nerve endings, the VZV gives rise to a simultaneous high density eruption of (chicken) pocks in the affected dermatome. As expected from the pathogenesis shingles is painful, unilateral and affects single or contiguous dermatomes.

Patients with shingles often have significant titres of VZV antibody at the time the rash is developing – thus reducing the possibility of dissemination. Despite this most patients with shingles do have a few chickenpoxes on their bodies: other patients, especially the immunosuppressed, may fail to prevent extensive secondary spread and generalized chickenpox may result.

Attacks of shingles may thus occur in anyone who has had an attack of chickenpox: in general attacks occur most often in the elderly or in the immunosuppressed, in those on cytotoxic drugs and in those who have malignancies (particularly Hodgkin's disease or chronic lymphatic leukaemia). Secondary and third attacks, although uncommon, are possible.

Although predominantly harboured in the sensory ganglia spread of infection may occur leading to motor nerve involvement with muscle paralysis.

Paporavirus infections

These viruses cause two main conditions:

(1) Progressive multifocal leukoencephalopathy which is a progressive demyelinating disease commonly affecting patients with underlying severe diseases, often of the reticuloendothelial system.

(2) Warts, of which there are five clinical types: verruca vulgaris (the common wart), verruca plana (planar warts often on the face, forehead, knees and shins), verruca plantaris (large painful plaques on the heels and soles), filiform warts (horny small excrescences usually on the face) and condyloma acuminata (genital warts). Given time most of these conditions would probably resolve spontaneously: treatment is usually by chemical destruction with agents such as trichloroacetic acid or podophylin.

Viral infections

Poxviruses

All poxviruses characteristically replicate in, and produce manifestations affecting, human skin.

There are four main conditions resulting from poxvirus infections.

(1) *Illnesses produced by animal infections which occasionally infect man*, usually causing hand lesions in animal handlers. Such diseases include cowpox, milkers' nodules (paravaccinia) and orf (which is a contagious granulomatous pustular dermatitis). Monkeypox and the related tanapox are occasionally acquired by humans in Africa.

(2) *Molluscum contagiosum* is usually spread by close contact. Waxy, hemispheric umbilicated papules occur, usually in the axilla or on the trunk. Treatment requires the destruction of each lesion.

(3) *Vaccinia* is a virus probably descended from cowpox. It is used for smallpox vaccination because it usually produces a trivial illness and it confers cross immunity to smallpox which lasts 3–5 years.

Complications of vaccination include an encephalitis and spread of infection which occurs in four main forms: generalized vaccinia, eczema vaccinatum, chronic progressive vaccinia and self inoculation of the virus to ectopic sites.

(4) *Smallpox* (variola). As man is the only known natural host for this virus and as prevention by vaccination is effective, smallpox has now been eradicated – although the virus still lurks in laboratories from where it has twice escaped. Smallpox had two clinically distinct variants, Variola major (classical smallpox), and the milder Variola minor (also known as alastrim). Infection was by droplet spread, from smallpox scabs or by fomites. The virus entered the body via the respiratory tract and subsequently spread to reticuloendothelial cells of many organs. The virus then entered the circulation (possibly causing a prodromal rash). A prodromal illness followed with fever, severe malaise, headache, backache, limb pains, and vomiting: this prodrome lasted 2–4 days and a maculopapular rash followed after the virus localized in the skin and mucous membranes. The rash then rapidly vesiculated and later crusted and scabs developed.

The differentiation between smallpox and chickenpox can be made rapidly by electron microscopy.

Vaccination with vaccinia virus gave useful protection against smallpox if given shortly after contact, as the incubation period of vaccinia is much shorter – usually 3 days.

Arenavirus infections

The name arenavirus refers to the sandlike granules seen within the virus on electron microscopy. Diseases produced include *Lymphocytic chorio-meningitis*, a disease that is only rarely transmitted to man from infected mice, and which produces an immune response mediated meningo-encephalitis, *Argentinian haemorrhagic fever* (Junin virus) and *Bolivian haemorrhagic fever* (Machupo virus) which both produce severe haemor-rhagic diseases. *Lassa fever* is an illness that appears to be transmitted primarily via the urine of infected rats and which causes a severe illness of high mortality. The incubation period is commonly 6–12 days (range 3–17 days). There is a non-specific insidious onset followed by severe prostration, membranous exudates or erosions on the pharynx, and often limb or back pains. Lassa fever probably occurs in bush areas throughout West Africa.

The laboratory diagnosis of all these illnesses, with the exception of lymphocytic choriomeningitis, requires high security facilities. Virus isol-ation, growth characteristics on cell cultures and serological tests all contribute towards identification of the virus involved.

Arbovirus infections

All these infections are transmitted to man by arthropod bites and in general produce either encephalitis or predominantly febrile illnesses, possibly with haemorrhagic accompaniments. Infections in Britain are invariably imported with the exception of *Louping ill* – a tick borne disease of sheep which occasionally causes an influenza-like syndrome or a meningoencephalitis in those exposed to infected sheep.

Particular arbovirus infections are usually given specific place names, but if infection with a particular virus is widely distributed non-geographical names are used. *Dengue* is a disease prevalent in South East Asia, India, the Pacific and the Caribbean: infection is mosquito trans-mitted (*Aedes aegypti*) and a 'breakbone fever' occurs – a severe febrile illness with excruciating musculoskeletal pains. *Dengue haemorrhagic fever* is a severe variant of Dengue, usually seen in children, consisting of additional shock and haemorrhages: it appears that the patients have altered immune responses induced by a previous attack of Dengue. *Yellow fever* occurs in certain areas of South America and Africa and, after a short incubation period, causes fever and jaundice possibly with haemorrhagic manifestation or renal involvement. Anicteric illnesses may occur.

Ebola virus infection

Small outbreaks of this infection have occurred in Northern Zaire and Southern Sudan in which the mortality was about 50%. The incubation period is 4–17 days after which there is a sudden onset of severe febrile illness with vomiting, diarrhoea and often a rash appears between days 4 and 7 of the illness. Haemorrhages may occur.

Enterovirus infections

The common pathogenic enteroviruses comprise coxsackieviruses (24 type A, 6 type B), echoviruses (30-plus serotypes) and polioviruses (three serotypes).

Coxsackievirus and echovirus infections

Many syndromes and diseases can result from the various coxsackie or echovirus infections. Asymptomatic infections are common. If illness results from infections the incubation period is often 7–14 days (2–35 possible). Most infections are acquired orally (either faecal-oral or from other host secretions) and the virus passes to reticuloendothelial tissue before spreading to various target organs.

Isolation of a particular virus from the throat or faeces does not confirm that virus as a pathogen: once an isolated virus has been identified, changes in relevant serum antibody levels have to be demonstrated to confirm that the host had reacted to that particular virus. There would be no change in antibody levels if a virus is non-invasive and pathogenically irrelevant. Isolation of an enterovirus from an unusual site for 'commensal presence' (cerebrospinal fluid or pericardium for example) is usually of pathogenic significance.

Identification of a virus by serological tests without prior culture typing is tedious and rarely justified unless a particular clinical syndrome is associated with only a few virus serotypes. In general neutralizing antibody tests are type specific and tend to persist, whereas complement fixing antibodies (which may not be serotype specific) fade within months.

With the exception of a few specific syndromes, coxsackievirus or echovirus infections may be suspected clinically if there is an acute febrile illness with evidence of multisystem involvement including meningism, myalgia, pneumonitis, enteric symptoms, glandular enlargement or skin rash, especially if contacts have had a similar self-limiting illness and if a septicaemia is unlikely.

'Non-specific' syndromes include aseptic meningitis, encephalitis, eye infections, febrile rashes which may be maculopapular or petechial (consider meningococcal septicaemia in the latter case), influenza-like illnesses, mild diarrhoea or vomiting, paralytic illnesses which are usually mild and transient, pharyngitis, pneumonitis and severe generalized disease especially in neonates. More specific syndromes include *Bornholm disease* (pleurodynia) usually caused by a Group B coxsackievirus and characterized by fever with severe myalgia, most marked in the chest or abdomen. *Hand, foot and mouth disease* usually caused by a Group A coxsackievirus causing fever and vesicles on the hands, feet and in the mouth. *Herpangina* usually caused by a Group A coxsackievirus resulting in fever, sore throat with a few greyish vesicles on the pharynx and *perimyocarditis* which is often caused by a Group B coxsackievirus.

Poliomyelitis

Polio may be caused by each of the three serotypes of poliovirus. Infection is usually faecal-oral, although droplet spread may occur as the virus is usually present in the pharynx a few days before and for up to 14 days after the onset of illness. The virus may be present in the stool for the period of illness and for a widely variable time thereafter.

Invasion of the central nervous system is apparently via the bloodstream, although experimental work has shown that the virus can travel along neural pathways. The essential lesion in the pathogenesis of polio is anterior horn cell and motor neuron necrosis. Other sites in the brain can be affected, particularly the motor nuclei of the brain stem causing bulbar paralysis.

After a 3–5 day incubation period a 'minor' or 'abortive' illness may result consisting of fever, mild headache and vague musculoskeletal pains lasting 4–5 days (corresponding to viraemia). The vast majority of patients recover but a minority develop the 'major' illness of paralytic polio with lower motor neuron type paralysis, which develops either directly or after a short latent period of 4–5 days. Thus there may be a biphasic pattern of illness.

In general the older the patient the more severe the paralysis, males are more often affected than females, the pregnant female is more severely affected than the non-pregnant female, previously traumatized or fatigued limbs are more affected, and Type 1 infections tend to cause more paralysis.

Diagnosis is by isolation of the virus from the stool or pharynx and by changes in antibody levels. Neutralizing antibodies are often present at the time paralysis occurs.

Treatment consists of absolute rest initially, later followed by physiotherapy with orthopaedic intervention as required. Intensive respiratory care is vital during paralysis involving respiratory muscles or the bulbar innervated muscles.

Prevention is either with injections of killed virus (Salk) or with the conventionally favoured live attenuated (Sabin) vaccine, in which three doses of vaccine containing attenuated strains of the three polio types are administered orally (with subsequent booster doses if necessary). Local gut immunity is also induced which minimizes possible invasion by wild (virulent) viruses. The relatively immediate interference with wild virus infection induced by prior vaccination with live virus vaccine is also useful in the termination of epidemics.

Hepatitis A ('infectious hepatitis')

Most infections occur in childhood: hepatitis A is usually acquired by the faecal-oral route (usually indirectly by food or water ingestion). The virus is present in the faeces for only a few days after the onset of jaundice, and it is likely that patients are most infectious *before* the onset of jaundice. Anicteric infections are common. The incubation period is between 15 and 40 days with a prodromal period (often shorter than that of hepatitis B) consisting of 2–3 days fever, nausea, vomiting and diarrhoea.

At present it is uncertain whether hepatic injury is mediated directly by the virus or host responses are of primary importance. Chronic infection does not occur although chronic persistent hepatitis or post hepatitic cholestasis may occur: both resolve given time and minimum interference.

Serological tests for hepatitis A are becoming widely available and, as occurred with hepatitis B, an epidemic of scientific papers will no doubt follow.

Pre-exposure prevention is possible with pooled human immunoglobulin. Protection lasts about six months and commences about two weeks after the injection.

Influenza

There are three strains of influenza virus. Minor changes in surface antigenic components of influenza occur constituting antigenic drift, whereas major changes produce abrupt antigenic shifts by which influenza A may give rise to 'new' epidemic virus strains to which whole populations may be vulnerable.

Influenza A tends to produce winter epidemics every two to three years. Influenza B in general produces a milder illness, whereas Influenza C in general produces a mild non-epidemic illness, usually in children. Spread is by droplet inhalation.

After an incubation period of 1–4 days there is an abrupt onset of fever, malaise, shivering, hacking cough, musculoskeletal pains, sore throat, nasal discharge and sneezing.

Influenza impairs the action of the cilia, alveolar macrophage activity is decreased and hypersecretion occurs: all of these favour secondary bacterial infection.

Diagnosis is by isolation of the virus or by serological tests of paired sera. Treatment of uncomplicated attacks of influenza is symptomatic. Prevention by vaccination will usually protect the majority of those at risk for about 3—6 months, providing the vaccine includes antigens derived from the current viral strains. Amantidine may also be useful prophylactically against influenza **A**.

Marburg virus infection

This highly lethal pantropic virus is perhaps better known as the causative agent of Green Monkey Disease: it is similar to, but serologically distinct from, Ebola virus. Various African-derived outbreaks have occurred in relation to vervet monkeys but the natural reservoir of infection is still obscure.

The incubation period is 3—9 days and illness is of an abrupt onset with headache, high fever, diarrhoea, a characteristic rash (a perifollicular, red, non-itching maculopapular eruption starting on the trunk), a bleeding tendency and signs of central nervous system involvement.

Measles

This is a highly infectious infection which causes manifestations in almost all susceptibles: immunity to a second attack is, however, lifelong. The mean incubation period to the appearance of a rash is 14 days, perhaps a little longer in adults. It is infectious during the prodromal period and for about 4—5 days after the onset of the rash.

Infection is usually by the respiratory route or via the conjunctivae: the virus then spreads to the regional lymph nodes and subsequently a primary viraemia (perhaps with a faint transient rash) spreads the virus to all lymphoid tissues. A secondary viraemia occurs and by the eleventh day prodromal symptoms of fever, catarrh and weepy eyes with conjunctivitis occur: the diagnostic Koplik's spots are usually evident.

The skin rash (exanthem) occurs in association with the development of reactive antibody and consists of a maculopapular blotchy rash which starts behind the ears and spreads downwards to the rest of the body.

A mucous membrane eruption occurs (an enanthem) which is usually noted on the buccal mucosa: these Koplik's spots are most prominent during the prodromal period and fade rapidly when the rash develops.

Respiratory involvement is usual resulting in a characteristic muffled cough.

Complications are most severe in the very old and the very young and include primary measles virus bronchitis or secondary bacterial pneumonia, otitis media, thrombocytopenia and haemorrhagic 'black' measles which possibly results from a severe vasculitis. An encephalitis may occur (in 0.1—0.2% of patients) with a peak period of onset at the sixth day of illness: it is thought to have an immunological causation as virus is not present in the brain tissue of those who die. *Subacute sclerosing panencephalitis* is

66

a rare, slowly progressive, almost invariably fatal illness consisting of deterioration of mental and physical cerebral function. The onset occurs years after the attack of measles: there are high levels of measles antibody in blood and cerebrospinal fluid, and the virus appears to be present in affected brain tissue. There is an association between high measles antibody levels and disseminated sclerosis but the significance of this is debated.

Confirmation of the diagnosis of measles is by isolation of the virus (possible but tedious): serology (especially by demonstration of changes in haemagglutination-inhibiting antibody) is more rapid and practical. Usually the clinical picture is diagnostic.

Measles vaccination is with a live attenuated virus. Human pooled immunoglobulin is useful prophylactically in at risk patients if given within 6–8 days of exposure.

Mumps (epidemic parotitis)

This virus is spread by droplets and has an affinity for glandular and nervous tissue, producing symptoms in approximately two-thirds of those infected. The incubation period is 16–18 days with infectivity from about three days before until about four days after parotid swelling. In classical 'parotitic' illness there is a brief prodrome of fever, myalgia and headache followed by parotid swelling which usually is, or becomes, bilateral: unilateral swelling occurs in about a quarter of those affected. Parotid swelling may be painful causing difficulty in mastication, which is not helped by the frequent occurrence of a dry mouth. The sublingual and submaxillary salivary glands may also be palpable. Parotid swelling has to be differentiated from lymph node enlargement: in the latter instance the groove behind the descending ramus of the mandible is not filled in.

Other possible manifestations of mumps virus infection may occur before, during, or after parotid swelling: they include meningoencephalitis, oophoritis, pancreatitis, myocarditis, nephritis, thyroiditis and arthritis. Epidydimo-orchitis with painful enlargement of the testis occurs in about a quarter of postpubertal males, this only rarely resulting in sterility even if orchitis is bilateral. Deafness, which is usually unilateral, may occur: mumps is a not uncommon cause of abrupt hearing loss in an uninflamed ear and the hearing loss is usually permanent.

Confirmation of diagnosis by serological tests is usually accomplished by finding complement fixing antibodies to either soluble (S) or viral (V) antigens. S antibodies are usually present after day seven of illness and peak in 2 weeks, whereas V antibodies are slower to appear (in 2–3 weeks) and persist for longer. A raised serum amylase, derived from parotid glands or pancreas, is found in 90% of patients with clinical parotitis.

Treatment is symptomatic with adequate analgesia. Steroids have been used for orchitis.

Parainfluenza infections

These viruses are important causes of lower respiratory diseases in children and upper respiratory diseases in adults. There are four main types, all of which are antigenically stable and replicate in respiratory epithelium without deeper invasion. Although there is some overlap in the syndromes produced, type 1 may produce croup (laryngotracheobronchitis) in children, type 2 may produce a similar milder illness, type 3 may cause pneumonia or bronchiolitis (particularly in those less than 6 months of age) and type 4 usually produces trivial respiratory illnesses.

All parainfluenza viruses are spread by person to person contact or by droplet spread, have short incubation periods and are highly infectious – although illness may not necessarily result from infection.

Clinical diagnosis of parainfluenza infection is impossible unless current epidemiological patterns are suggestive. Diagnosis is by isolation of the virus or by serological tests.

Rabies

This virus is neurotropic and is usually transmitted by the bite of a rabid dog or cat and, in humans at least, is almost invariably fatal once neurological symptoms develop. Infection may be acquired from bites of other animals.

Rabies, at the time of writing, is not present in British wildlife and human infections are all imported. The main reservoir of European rabies is the fox.

In general the virus is present in the saliva of affected dogs or cats 3–5 days before the onset of illness (exceptionally up to two weeks before illness).

The incubation period of human rabies is variable, usually being 2–8 weeks but incubation periods of longer than two years have been thought to occur. After a bite from a rabid animal the virus multiplies locally and travels to the central nervous system via the peripheral nerves. There follows a 2–4 day prodrome. Fever, headache, nausea and a sense of apprehension are non-specific symptoms, and a more specifically suggestive symptom is pain or paraesthesiae in the bitten area. The ensuing illness may be 'furious' rabies, with central nervous system irritability manifested by excitation, convulsions and hypersensitivity to various stimuli. Dysphagia with painful spasms (hydrophobia) may be precipitated by the taste, smell or thought of water or food; the resulting choking may cause severe apnoea and cyanosis. Lacrimation, salivation and sweating reflect enhanced sympathetic nervous activity. A preterminal paralytic stage follows – death usually occurring 2–6 days after the onset of symptoms, the patient usually having been conscious and alert throughout. Occasionally a

68

purely paralytic rabies results with ascending paralysis and sensory disturbances.

Although human to human transmission is theoretically possible (especially to medical and nursing attendants) it is as yet unrecorded.

Diagnosis is by:

(1) observation of the biting animal for signs of rabies (if a dog or cat, for ten days),

(2) examination of tissue obtained from the biting animal – light microscopy of brain tissue may reveal intracytoplasmic inclusion bodies (Negri bodies) which, if detected, are diagnostic,

(3) fluorescent antibody tests,

(4) laboratory animal inoculation.

Treatment of a potentially infected bite needs the rapid assessment of the degree of risk followed, if necessary, by urgent therapy including adequate wound toilet, administration of immune serum (both locally and systemically) and vaccination. Coincidental tetanus immunization may also be indicated. The biting animal, if obtainable, should be observed.

Detailed recommendations regarding rabies prevention and treatment are given in the WHO Sixth Report of the expert committee on rabies; WHO Technical Report Services 523, (1973) or in the DHSS Memorandum on Rabies, (1977). Expert local advice should be obtained.

Respiratory syncytial virus infections

This virus causes syncytium formation (a large cell with many nuclei) in tissue culture, hence the name. It causes lower respiratory tract infections in infancy and early childhood, notably bronchiolitis and pneumonia: it may also cause a common cold syndrome. Transmission is by respiratory secretions and the incubation period is probably about 4–5 days. Most individuals are infected early in life despite the transplacental transfer of (IgG) antibodies – presumably the virus flourishes in the respiratory tract because of absence of local immunity. Typically the mucous membranes of nose and throat are involved, possibly with spread to the trachea, bronchioles and lung parenchyma. Secondary atelectasis and infection may occur.

Diagnosis is by isolation of the virus (which may be difficult as it is labile and often difficult to culture) or by demonstration of significant antibody changes. Immunofluorescent studies of respiratory tract secretions are also useful.

Treatment for the syndromes produced is described in Chapter 8. Vaccine development is in progress but this may be difficult as allergic mechanisms may contribute to pathogenicity – and vaccines might produce an allergic state.

Rhinovirus infections

These viruses are a frequent cause of the common cold. There are over one hundred antigenically distinct serotypes and thus the development of an overall vaccine is improbable.

The viruses exhibit optimal growth at 33–35°C, and as general body temperature is 37°C manifestations of infection remain substantially localized in the cooler nasal passages, where they produce hyperaemia and oedema of the nasal passage mucous membranes with out-pouring of serous fluid and mucus.

Virus shedding is mainly from the nose and only to a lesser extent in saliva and other respiratory secretions. Infection is spread primarily by bodily contact, usually by hand to hand contact. Aerosol production and kissing (under controlled conditions!) have been shown to be an inefficient method of spread. It appears that subsequent transfer of infection to the nose (perhaps via the conjunctivae) is by fingers of the future sufferer.

The incubation period is 1–4 days, after which an illness of about seven days duration ensues with upper respiratory tract symptoms of rhinorrhoea, nasal obstruction and sneezing. Usually there are no other symptoms or signs: fever, if it occurs, is not marked and the cough is not hacking in nature as in influenza.

Diagnosis of rhinovirus infection is clinically difficult: the virus has to be isolated from the nasal discharge.

Rotavirus infections

This virus is a common cause of diarrhoea, particularly in infants.

Rubella (German measles) infection

This virus is probably spread by the respiratory route and, after multiplication in the respiratory epithelium and regional lymph nodes, a viraemia occurs which disseminates the virus. The resulting rash is probably caused by an antigen–antibody reaction rather than by direct viral invasion of skin vascular endothelium.

The incubation period is commonly 18 days and a patient is usually infectious up to 7 days before and up to 5 days after illness. Immunity to a second attack is usually lifelong although confirmed rubella has occurred in those with natural or vaccine-induced immunity.

Complications include arthralgia and arthritis of fingers, wrists and knees, most notably in young adult females. Rarer complications include encephalitis, thrombocytopenia and neuritis.

Viral infections

Congenital rubella is produced by foetal infection consequent to maternal viraemia: affected infants excrete the virus for a long time after birth and thus pose a considerable infection risk. About 16% of infants have major defects at birth following maternal rubella in the first three months of pregnancy. The incidence and type of induced defects are related to the age of the foetus at the time of infection.

Congenital rubella may affect:

(1) *The eye* − causing cataracts, retinopathy, microphthalmia or glaucoma.
(2) *The cardiovascular system* − causing patent ductus arteriosus, ventricular septal defects or pulmonary stenosis.
(3) *The ear* − causing deafness.
(4) *Other tissues* − possibly resulting in thrombocytopenic purpura, hepatosplenomegaly, hepatitis, central nervous system defects or bone lesions.

Serological diagnosis is most simply performed by assay of the haemagglutination inhibition antibody titres (HAI) which rise within 1−2 days of the rash, peak within 6−12 days, then fade and persist at low levels thereafter. Complement fixing antibodies appear about 7−10 days after the rash and peak 1−2 months later, thereafter fading slowly: complement fixing antibodies tests are useful if serological testing has been delayed for any reason.

Prevention is with a live attenuated vaccine which produces HAI antibodies in 90−98% of seronegative vaccinees. Vaccination may produce a mild rubella-like illness. Ideally all females should be rubella immune prior to conception (the local laboratory should be consulted to discover the level of HAI that is considered to represent immunity). If pregnant and non-immune they should be offered vaccination after delivery. Females should not be pregnant or become so within eight to twelve weeks of vaccination. The suggested action to be taken if a pregnant woman is suspected of having rubella or to have been in contact with rubella is detailed in Chapter 14.

Bacteriophages

These are viruses that infect bacteria and identification of such virus infection may accurately label the precise bacteria responsible for a particular infection. For example, the bacteria *Staph. aureus* of a particular phage type (71) may cause toxic epidermal necrolysis.

Certain bacteriophages can contribute to bacterial pathogenicity by evoking the production of exotoxin − examples include the diphtheria toxin and the erythrogenic toxin produced by certain strains of *Strep. pyogenes*.

Slow virus infections (Table 2)

Slow viruses do not cause an acute illness, but rather cause infection characterized by a long incubation period and a slowly progressive course. Diseases possibly caused by, or associated with, slow virus infection include motor neurone disease, Parkinson's disease, rheumatoid arthritis, ulcerative colitis, Creutzfeldt–Jakob disease (a progressive neurological disease), Kuru (a demyelinating disease of cannibals) and Crohn's disease.

THERAPY OF VIRAL INFECTIONS

As can be seen from this brief review of the major pathogenic viruses, therapy is in most cases supportive, with isolation of the patient if appropriate. At present antiviral chemotherapy is not available for most viral infections and all antibacterial drugs are of course ineffective.

In future genetic engineering may make large scale production of interferon possible: interferon blocks viral invasion and secondary spread of most viruses within a host. Interferon or similar broad spectrum antiviral agents are no doubt drugs of great potential.

Suggested further reading

Evans, A.S. (1976). *Viral Infections of Humans.* (New York: John Wiley and Sons)

4
Fungal infections

Fungi include *moulds* which have long filamentous hyphae which form networks (mycelia), *yeasts* which are single celled fungi that reproduce by budding, *yeast-like fungi* which may exist partly as yeasts and partly as filaments, and *Dimorphic fungi* which exist as filaments or yeasts, depending on circumstances. They are widely distributed in nature and some species may be commensal organisms: it follows from this that identification of a fungus from various specimens is not necessarily of pathogenic significance.

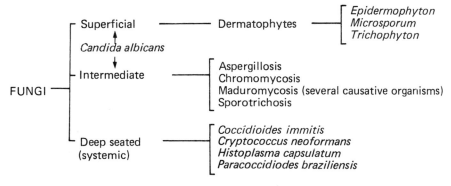

Figure 15   A classification of the major pathogenic fungi

Fungal illnesses are usually produced if the number of attacking fungal organisms is sufficiently high or if the host is vulnerable to attack: vulnerability may be caused by many factors but defective cell mediated immunity seems to be particularly relevant.

Certain fungi exhibit marked tissue tropism, whilst others tend to produce marked delayed type hypersensitivity reactions which may contribute towards the disease manifestations. The diagnosis of fungal infections is made by direct examination of tissue sections, scrapings or excreta, and by culture.

SUPERFICIAL FUNGAL INFECTIONS

These are relatively common and are caused by various organisms which thrive on, and remain localized in the keratin in hair, nails or skin. One suspects a fungal infection in any asymmetrical, well defined, scaley, inflamed area, especially if there are small vesicles or pustules at the perimeter.

Infections are usually, albeit loosely, referred to as Tinea of various sites.

T. barbae causes an eruption of the beard area. Griseofulvin is the treatment of choice.

T. capitis mainly affects children and may produce semi-bald, greyish patches on the scalp often with broken hairs. Griseofulvin given by mouth may be used in association with topical applications of antifungal agents.

T. corporis (circinata) classically causes ring-like lesions with raised borders. For localized lesions miconazole or clotrimazole cream or lotion should be applied. For extensive or persistent disease griseofulvin may be required.

T. cruris occurs in the groin area and forms an abnormal area extending around the genitals and the adjacent inner thighs. Lesions are often complicated by dampness, maceration and secondary infection with bacteria or candida. Griseofulvin is usually necessary: topical treatment tends to be messy and ineffective unless the infection is very limited.

T. pedis (athlete's foot) is a very common infection of the interdigital spaces of the feet. Lesions are often macerated and have scaling borders: vesicles may be seen. For alleviation, and hopefully cure, good foot hygiene is essential. The interdigital spaces must be well dried after bathing, macerated skin gently rubbed away and an antifungal dusting powder applied. 'Airy' permeable footware is helpful. Whitfields ointment may also be useful. If all else fails griseofulvin is effective.

T. unguium (of the nails) occurs more often in the feet than in the hands. The nails become thickened and dull in appearance. Treatment, if necessary, requires griseofulvin until all the infected nail has grown out: for fingernails this may be 6–12 months and even longer for toenails.

T. versicolor is common in young adults, and produces an unsightly mottled appearance of the skin. The patches are round or oval and vary in size from a few millimetres to a few centimetres, and commonly look like 'pale raindrops' as they do not tan after exposure to the sun. Without exposure to the sun they may be darker than the surrounding skin (hence versicolor). Treatment, if necessary, can be with topical selenium.

Tinea infections are colloquially called ringworm as the infections often produce a widening ring with a brownish red periphery with scaling and perhaps with vesicles or pustules. Ringworm is the only fungal disease readily transmitted from man to man. Occasionally extensive pustular abscesses called kerions may occur. Superficial fungal infection in one situation may produce a sympathetic eruption in unaffected areas elsewhere.

INTERMEDIATE FUNGAL INFECTIONS

These include those infections which tend to remain localized but which may spread given suitable circumstances.

Aspergillus organisms are common in the environment and as commensals: they may produce various illness patterns ranging from hypersensitivity reactions with bronchospasm (with associated immediate type skin sensitivity and possibly eosinophilia) to progressive invasive disease. Infection is commonly acquired by the respiratory route and fungus balls (mycetoma) may occur in lung cavities − especially in tuberculous cavities. Locally invasive disease may result and metastatic spread may occur particularly to the kidney and brain.

Candida (Monilia) infection usually results from infection with *Candida albicans*, but other species of Candida may produce illness. Candida usually affects vulnerable patients including the very young or the very old, those with diabetes, the immunodeficient, those on antibacterial therapy, and those with altered hormonal states including pregnancy. Resulting illnesses include stomatitis, pharyngitis possibly leading to oesophagitis, vaginal discharge, some nappy rashes, intertrigo (lesions in the skinfolds of the obese or copiously perspiring) and paronychia. More serious disease can result in patients with severe underlying disease − chronic mucocutaneous candidiasis may occur in immunodeficiency states, disseminated infection may occur in the seriously ill and endocarditis (with characteristically large emboli) in intravenous drug receivers. Torulopsis, a yeast, is similar to Candida and notably causes urinary tract infections in the catheterized.

All the following fungal diseases are not indigenous to Britain with the exception of *Cryptococcus neoformans*.

Chloromycosis produces a chronic itching cauliflower-like ulceration, usually on the legs.

Maduromycosis (Madura foot) has several causative organisms and probably results from traumatic implantation of organisms into the foot, resulting in swelling and sinuses draining granular pus.

Sporotrichosis has a wide geographical distribution. Organisms are inoculated via thorns or splinters and about 2 weeks later a chancre-like lesion results with a chain of abscesses developing along draining lymphatic channels.

DEEP FUNGAL INFECTIONS

These infections commonly exhibit systemic spread.

Coccidioides immitis occurs on the American continent and, in a small proportion of those infected, causes a chronic granulomatous disease in the lungs with possible dissemination. Hypersensitivity reactions may result leading to erythema nodosum, erythema multiforme or arthralgia.

Cryptococcus neoformans (previously known as Torula) may produce illnesses varying from inapparent respiratory infections to disseminated infection affecting virtually any organ, but particularly affecting the central nervous system where it causes a subacute or chronic meningitis. Infection is by inhalation of dust contaminated by bird faeces. Although it may affect normal individuals, cryptococcal infection should be particularly suspected in any immunocompromised patient who develops a non-bacterial meningitis.

Histoplasma capsulatum is similar to *Coccidioides immitis* but has a wider geographical distribution. Infection is derived from soil, particularly that contaminated with bird or bat faeces. Human infection seems to be via the respiratory tract, causing acute respiratory infections, chronic cavitating lung disease or a progressive disseminated infection.

Paracoccidioides braziliensis (South American blastomycosis) causes a chronic progressive granulomatous disease which frequently attacks mucous membranes and lymphatic tissues.

THERAPY OF FUNGAL INFECTIONS

Superficial infections usually respond to topical or local therapy in association with attention to predisposing factors, if any. In conditions where local applications are ineffective, systemic therapy may have to be undertaken. Intermediate and deep infections usually require systemic therapy.

Amphotericin B is usually administered by local application or intravenously. It has a wide spectrum of activity against fungal infections, including *Candida albicans*, and most of the deep fungal infections including *Cryptococcus neoformans* and *Histoplasma capsulatum*. It acts on the sterol-containing cytoplasmic membrane and, as human cells also possess sterols, there are problems with toxicity when amphotericin is given systemically. For local administration there are various preparations including creams, ointments, lotions, suppositories, pessaries and lozenges. During intravenous infusions there may be fever, headache, nausea and vomiting and thrombophlebitis. Nephrotoxicity and anaemia are predictable side effects depending on the dosage and duration of therapy. Thus systemic amphotericin B is only given to treat serious infections.

Clotrimazole and micronazole. The former has a wide range of activity but its common usage, at present, is topically as it is active against *both* candida and cutaneous tinea infections, this being one of its major advantages. Miconazole can be given systemically to treat immediate and deep fungal infections. Both clotrimazole and miconazole are available as creams, the former is also available as a spray or powder and the latter in tablet form.

5-Fluorocytosine, although of low toxicity, has a relatively narrow spectrum and is most useful for disseminated candida and cryptococcal infections; when used in the treatment of cryptococcal infection there is synergism with amphotericin B. The two drugs can also be used in combination against fungi for which 5-fluorocytosine alone would not be appropriate. 5-fluorocytosine can be given in tablet form or intravenously. It has been given intrathecally.

Griseofulvin is a relatively non-toxic drug active against cutaneous tinea infections. It accumulates in keratin and has to be given for long periods until infected material has been shed. It has no useful activity against candida, cryptococci or the deep fungi. Oral therapy depends on body size, varying from 500 mg daily for small patients to 1000 mg daily for large patients.

Natamycin is a relatively non-toxic drug with a wide spectrum of antifungal activity. Its main use is against candida and cutaneous tinea infections. It is particularly useful for the treatment of both the common causes of vaginal discharge as it is effective against candida and *Trichomonas vaginalis* (a protozoa) – although a definitive diagnosis followed by organism specific therapy would probably be more efficacious. Natamycin can be given topically, orally or as an aerosol (for pulmonary infections).

Nystatin. Although this drug has a wide spectrum of activity *in vitro* its major use is in topical treatment of *Candida albicans* infections of skin, vagina, mouth and bowel. It is available in creams, ointments, pessaries, suspensions and tablet forms.

Tolnaftate is used for tinea infections as a cream, solution or powder.

Whitfield's ointment contains both benzoic and salicylic acids. It is cheap but messy and is effective against cutaneous tinea infections. The same comments apply to Castellani's paint and potassium permanganate.

Other antifungal agents are available including econazole, chlorophenesin and many broad-spectrum antiseptics.

Suggested further reading

Wilcocks, C. and Manson-Bahr (1974). *Manson's Tropical Diseases.* Section 8; Diseases caused by Fungi. (London: Baillière Tindall)

5
Protozoal infections

Protozoa are single celled organisms in which one cell is capable of performing all functions necessary for an independent existence: they may be considered to be the lowest form of animal life. They are often motile by virtue of pseudopodia formation or by the possession of flagellae. Some protozoa have the capability to form thick walled resting cells (cysts) which ensure persistence and which may be a vehicle for spread of infection.

Most pathogenic protozoa are vulnerable to chemotherapy.

Figure 16 lists the major pathogenic protozoa.

AMOEBIC INFECTIONS

Under normal circumstances *Entamoeba histolytica* is the only pathogenic amoeba. It is usually, but not always, acquired in tropical or subtropical regions by ingestion of cysts in contaminated food or water; such cysts can survive in a suitable environment for about 30 days. In symptomatic infections the amoebae initially invade the gut wall of the appendix region, caecum and ascending colon; they then penetrate the mucosa and submucosa forming abscesses which then rupture into the gut lumen forming ulcers with raised undermined edges and necrotic centres. Such lesions may occur distally (and become visible on sigmoidoscopy). Classically, there is a slow onset of large bowel type diarrhoea which may be blood streaked.

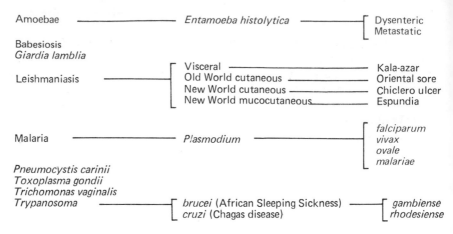

Figure 16 Major pathogenic Protozoa

Metastatic spread of the invasive amoebae may occur with or without colonic symptoms or signs, commonly manifesting as abscess(es) which usually occur in the right lobe of the liver. Symptoms include fever, sweats, pain in the right upper abdomen, and right sided rib tenderness. Occasionally metastatic spread may occur to other organs such as the lung and brain.

Diagnosis of infection is by demonstration of either the amoebae themselves or their cysts in a freshly passed stool, or by demonstration of the amoebae in scrapes or aspirates of abscess pus (which resembles anchovy sauce). Such examinations may need to be repeated and concentration methods applied. Serological tests, including fluorescent antibody and complement fixation tests, are particularly useful if there is extra-intestinal spread. Amoebic pus, unlike bacterial pus, does *not* contain a large number of polymorphonuclear cells, a point of diagnostic importance.

Treatment is with high dose metronidazole which is usually effective, but emetine hydrochloride or chloroquine are also of therapeutic value. Drainage is only occasionally necessary if liver abscesses are very large.

Rarely other amoebae (*Hartmanella* and *Naegleria*) cause a meningoencephalitis with turbid cerebrospinal fluid containing the amoebae. It is acquired by swimming in contaminated water. Treatment is with amphotericin B.

Balantidium coli produces an illness similar to *Entamoeba histolytica*: it is commonly acquired from pigs and treatment is with metronidazole, diodohydroxyonin or tetracycline.

BABESIOSIS

This is a rare disease transmitted by the bite of certain ticks. The parasite becomes intracellular in erythrocytes causing haemolysis and fever.

Protozoal infections

GIARDIA LAMBLIA

This flagellate parasite resides in the glandular crypts of the duodenal and jejunal mucosa. If infection is extensive upper small bowel function is disrupted and a malabsorptive-type diarrhoea results with frequent pale stools and occasionally there is gross steatorrhoea. In the tropics infection with *Giardia lamblia* is not uncommon (up to 25% of the population in some regions) and it is a very common cause of persistent travellers' diarrhoea in those who have visited the tropics.

Transmission is by ingestion of cysts which are viable for about three months in suitable damp environments.

Diagnosis is by demonstration of the parasites themselves in duodenal aspirates or more commonly by finding cysts in the stool.

Treatment is with metronidazole or mepacrine.

LEISHMANIASIS

These protozoa are intracellular parasites of the reticuloendothelial system and are usually transmitted by sandflies.

Visceral leishmaniasis

Visceral leishmaniasis is also known as Kala-azar (Hindi for black illness) and is caused by *L. donovani*, an organism widely distributed in tropical and subtropical Asia and Africa, the Mediterranean and tropical South America. Man to man transmission occurs via sandflies but in certain regions an intermediate host is present. The incubation period is usually about three to six months but the range is much wider. Illness starts with irregular malaise, headache, fever (possibly with two spikes per day), splenomegaly, hepatomegaly and hyperpigmentation (hence the name). There may be anaemia, leukopenia, thrombocytopenia and hyperglobulin-aemia secondary to hypersplenism and immune mechanisms. Without treatment clinical disease is usually fatal.

Diagnosis is by demonstration of the parasite in macrophages and tissue obtained from splenic puncture, sternal marrow, lymph nodes or liver biopsy. Serological tests, including complement fixation tests, are also used.

Treatment is with sodium stibogluconate: prevention is by elimination of the sandflies or their intermediate vector if any.

Old World cutaneous leishmaniasis (Oriental sore)

This superficial infection is found in Mediterranean areas, South West and Central Asia and North Africa. A reddish papule with crusting occurs at the

81

site of organism inoculation, often the face. A shallow ulcer with sharp raised edges may also result. Spontaneous healing would eventually occur leaving a depressed, depigmented scar but treatment with sodium stibogluconate or local heat may be necessary if the lesions are disfiguring.

Diagnosis is by demonstration of the organism.

New World cutaneous leishmaniasis (Chiclero ulcer)

This is usually caused by *L. mexicana* and results in non-metastasizing ulcers or swellings which invade directly, but which usually heal spontaneously.

New World mucocutaneous leishmaniasis (espundia)

This is caused by *L. braziliensis*. It is found in Central and South America. The organisms metastasize to mucous membranes and mucocutaneous junctions particularly of the nose, larynx, pharynx and face leading to ulceration, extensive necrosis and polyp formation: deformity may be extensive. Sodium stibogluconate is effective.

MALARIA (Figure 17)

Human infection is caused by four malarial parasites – *Plasmodium falciparum* causes malignant tertian* malaria, *Plasmodium vivax* and *Plasmodium ovale* both cause benign tertian malaria, and *Plasmodium malariae* causes benign quartan† malaria.

Parasites (sporozoites) of all species are injected by the bite of a female anopheline mosquito and then pass to the human liver where they divide by multiple asexual reproductions (schizogony), the reproductive rate being most marked in falciparum malaria. After a variable period of time parasites (merozoites) are released into the blood thus terminating the primary liver cycle (also known as the primary exoerythrocytic cycle). The released parasites then enter erythrocytes and undergo a second period of asexual reproduction (erythrocytic schizogony) and are subsequently released to invade other erythrocytes. Other parasites change into sexual forms (gametocytes) which are released into the blood, and if this blood is sucked up by a female anopheline mosquito a period of sexual reproduction follows and sporozoites are formed. The mosquito–human liver–human erythrocyte cycle is thereby completed.

However there is a therapeutically important 'side-cycle': *Plasmodium vivax*, *Plasmodium ovale* and possibly *Plasmodium malariae* parasites,

---

*Tertian means every third day.
†Quartan means every fourth day.

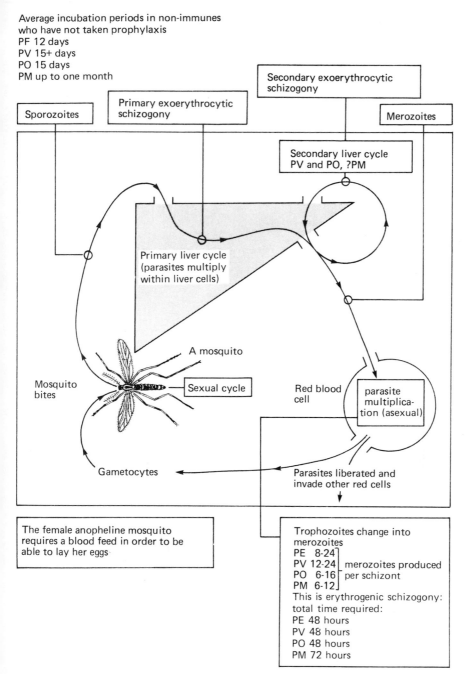

Average incubation periods in non-immunes
who have not taken prophylaxis
PF 12 days
PV 15+ days
PO 15 days
PM up to one month

Secondary exoerythrocytic
schizogony

Sporozoites

Primary exoerythrocytic
schizogony

Merozoites

Secondary liver cycle
PV and PO, ?PM

Primary liver cycle
(parasites multiply
within liver cells)

A mosquito

Mosquito
bites

Sexual cycle

Red blood
cell

parasite
multiplica-
tion (asexual)

Gametocytes

Parasites liberated and
invade other red cells

The female anopheline mosquito
requires a blood feed in order to be
able to lay her eggs

Trophozoites change into
merozoites
PE 8-24 ⎤
PV 12-24 ⎟ merozoites produced
PO 6-16 ⎟ per schizont
PM 6-12 ⎦
This is erythrogenic schizogony:
total time required:
PE 48 hours
PV 48 hours
PO 48 hours
PM 72 hours

Figure 17   The life cycle of malaria: the inner area is the simplified version and the
outer areas are the complex version. PF = *Plasmodium falciparum*, PV =
Plasmodium vivax, PO = *Plasmodium ovale* and PM = *Plasmodium malariae*

83

Table 3 The drug treatment of an acute attack of malaria

Drug	Major toxicity	Curative oral dosage for adults	Oral for child	Intravenous	Other points
Chloroquine	Uncommon, pruritus, headache, visual disturbances	600 mg at 0 hours 300 mg at 6 hours 300 mg at 30 hours 300 mg at 54 hours (1.5 g in total)	10 mg/kg, 5 mg/kg, 5 mg/kg, 5 mg/kg with same time intervals	Initially 300 mg in at least 300 ml N saline over at least 30 min	Resistance a problem in some areas. Safe in pregnancy. Suppositories of 150–300 mg base are available. IV causes hypotension. Do not use IV in children
Quinine	Cinchonism: nausea, vomiting, tinnitus, vertigo	650 mg 8 hourly for 10–14 days	Less than 1 yr 162 mg b.d. 1–3 yrs 162 mg t.d.s. 4–6 yrs 325 mg b.d. 7–10 yrs 325 mg t.d.s.	600 mg in at least 100 ml 5% glucose slowly, repeat 8 hourly if necessary	Use in chloroquine resistance. Excreted by the kidney and metabolized by the liver. If haemolysis occurs treatment must be stopped. Ideal serum level 5–10 mg/litre. Quinine followed by Fansidar gives a cure rate of about 90% in chloroquine-resistant *Plasmodium falciparum* infections
Pyrimethamine					A back-up drug only in chloroquine resistance
Trimethoprim					A back-up drug only in chloroquine resistance
Fansidar	Sulphonamide side-effects	2–3 tabs.			Probably in third place (to quinine or chloroquine).
Mefloquine					Further evaluation awaited
Primaquine	Haemolytic anaemias in glucose-6-phosphate deficiency states	7.5 mg of base b.d. for 14 days	0.25 mg/kg/day for 14 days		Use after chloroquine treatment to eradicate secondary exoerythrocytic stage

Do not forget supportive care, aspirin, sponging and fanning. Accurate fluid balance is essential.

after their initial release from the liver, can return to and multiply within the liver *without having to pass through erythrocytes* (this 'side-cycle' constitutes secondary exoerythrocytic schizogony). Antimalarial treatment such as chloroquine, which primarily attacks the intra-erythrocytic parasites, will therefore not eradicate these infections and an additional drug, usually primaquine, has to be given to eradicate the secondary hepatic cycle. *Plasmodium falciparum* can be cured with chloroquine alone as these parasites cannot re-enter the liver.

Symptoms of malaria usually consist of abrupt onset of fever, headache, rigors, and myalgia. Splenomegaly occurs in about half of patients with acute malaria. In an acute attack there is usually *no* temporal pattern to the fever, but later, when synchronized erythrocytic schizogony and synchronized release of parasites from the erythrocytes occurs, regular paroxysms of fever may occur. (In any case the diagnosis should have been made and treatment instituted before fever patterns have emerged.)

Diagnosis is by examination of appropriately stained blood films.

Prevention can be achieved with a number of drugs (Chapter 14); the drugs used for treatment of an acute attack are detailed in Table 3. In chloroquine resistant areas Fansidar (a combination of sulphadoxine and pyrimethamine) is useful for prevention or treatment but quinine is usually used for an acute attack.

The distribution of malaria and chloroquine-resistant *P. falciparum* is given in Figures 34 and 35, in Chapter 10.

PNEUMOCYSTIS CARINII

This is a widely distributed organism of almost zero pathogenicity except in patients with defective immune responses, haematological malignancies or severe malnutrition. Active infection usually results in an interstitial pneumonia with the chest X-ray showing bilateral infiltrates.

Diagnosis is by demonstration of the organism in sputum, in tracheal aspirates or in lung biopsy.

Treatment is with pentamidine. Co-trimoxazole may have a role to play in both treatment and prophylaxis.

TOXOPLASMA GONDII

This parasite is of worldwide distribution. Infection is transmitted by ingestion or droplet spread from members of the cat family which are usually the definitive hosts. Most infections are sub-clinical but in acquired toxoplasmosis there is an acute inflammatory reaction to the localized parasites and to parasitaemia. Several illnesses may result, a febrile or non-febrile lymphadenitis, or a pyrexial illness: a macular rash may occur in each. A potentially fatal meningoencephalomyelitis may occur, especially in immunocompromised hosts. Myocarditis, hepatitis and 'atypical' pneumonias also occur.

Congenital infection occurs when a mother *first acquires* toxoplasmosis during pregnancy. A *previously infected* mother suppresses further infection and the foetus is not affected. An affected child may be damaged in several ways: hydrocephalus, calcified (usually cerebral) granulomas, choroidoretinitis in 90% (the major clinical clue) and epilepsy constitute the tetrad of Sabin. The following may also occur: anaemia, microcephalus, focal necroses of various organs, fever, rash, jaundice, purpura, hepatosplenomegaly and mental retardation.

The diagnosis may be suspected if there are atypical lymphocytes in the blood film, and is confirmed if the organism can be visualized or isolated on biopsy. However, serological tests are commonly used to substantiate the diagnosis. The Toxoplasma dye test is usually positive at a titre of greater than 1:1000 in acute infection, but significant changes in titre are needed to confirm acute infection. In the absence of an acute illness this test is of limited value except as a population screening test. The complement fixation test becomes positive later than the dye test, but becomes negative more quickly, thus indicating a fairly recent infection. IgM and IgG titres are useful, IgM is raised in the first week of an acute infection and peaks at one month.

Treatment is with a combination of sulphadiazine and pyrimethamine, or with spiramycin.

TRICHOMONAS VAGINALIS

This infection is primarily a sexually transmitted disease. For clinical details see Chapter 11.

TRYPANOSOMIASIS

There are two main illnesses produced:

(1) *T. cruzi (Chagas disease)*
This occurs in Central America, Mexico, Costa Rica and South America. It is transmitted by the faeces of blood-sucking bugs which are scratched into the skin. After an incubation period of 7–14 days, an erythematous indurated area at the site of skin infection occurs (the chagoma) in association with an acute illness consisting of fever, headache, local and generalized oedema, hepatosplenomegaly, signs of heart involvement, or meningoencephalitis. Intense periorbital oedema, chemosis and lacrimal adenitis constitutes Romana's signs. The mortality rate is 10% or less.

Decades later, involvement of 'hollow organs' becomes evident, in the heart producing heart failure or heart block, in the colon and oesophagus leading to peristaltic malfunction and distension.

Diagnosis is by demonstration of the organism which is continually present in the blood during the acute stage, in the chronic stage the organism is intermittently present. Biopsy, culture and serology including complement fixation testing may be useful.

No curative treatment is available.

(2) *African Sleeping Sickness*

This disease is transmitted by various tsetse flies (*Glossinia*) which are found in rural areas of the savannah, particularly in relationship to water-holes. At the site of the insect bite a painless, non-suppurative lesion a few inches in diameter may occur (the trypanosomal chancre). Subsequently spread occurs via blood and lymph and is associated with irregular remittant fever, a transient annular erythematous rash in whites, headache, itching, hepatosplenomegaly, and lymph node enlargement particularly of the posterior cervical triangle (Winterbottom's sign). Later central nervous system invasion occurs which, if untreated, leads to a chronic meningoencephalitis resulting in slow speech, apathy, tremors, psychosis, unsteady gait, coma and death.

There are two types of African Sleeping Sickness: *T. gambiense* is more common in West Africa and produces, after an incubation period of up to several years, a slow onset of a slowly progressive disease, whereas *T. rhodesiense* produces a more abrupt onset of a more rapidly progressive illness after an incubation period of 5–21 days. *T. rhodesiense* is more common in East and East Central Africa.

Diagnosis in general is by visualization of the organism in stained blood films, from the chancre, from lymph nodes or from the cerebrospinal fluid. Animal inoculation is also useful as are serological tests, particularly on cerebrospinal fluid. Blood IgM levels are usually markedly raised.

Treatment is with suramin, melarsoprol or pentamidine.

Suggested further reading

Wilcocks, C. and Manson-Bahr, P.E.C. (1974). *Manson's Tropical Diseases. Section 1; Diseases caused by Protozoa.* (London: Baillière Tindall)

6
Worm infections

Serious worm infections are uncommon in western countries but in other parts of the world, such as Africa, the Middle and Far East, infection is common and much ill health results. Most worm infections have both scientific and popular names (Figure 18).

There are three major divisions of pathogenic worm infections – the Cestodes, Nematodes and the Trematodes. Worms that inhabit the gastro-intestinal tract may be diagnosed by requesting stool examination for ova, cysts or for the parasites themselves.

For detailed information concerning exact geographical locations and treatments the reader is referred to specialist texts. For clarity some of the diagrams in this chapter illustrate autoinfection – other humans would be infected by material derived from excretory products of a host. In British patients who have not been abroad threadworm, ascaris and tapeworm infections are the most likely worm infections to present clinically. If a patient has 'passed a worm as large as an earthworm' it is either an ascaris or a tapeworm: in the latter instance the worm will be segmented.

CESTODES

All except hydatid disease will respond to niclosamide.

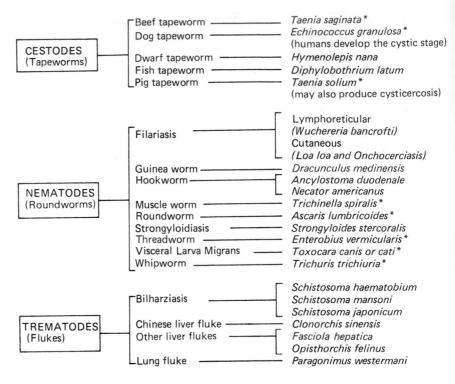

Figure 18   A classification of the major pathogenic worms, with their common names

*Can be acquired in Britain: the remainder are almost always imported

Beef tapeworm

Man is the primary host.*

Diagnosis is by identification of the eggs or examination of an expelled worm.

Dog tapeworm

Man is an accidental intermediate host and hydatid disease results. Hydatid cysts are produced in the liver in 65% and in the lung in 25% of patients, but the cysts may develop in any organ. Hydatid cysts cause pressure

*The primary or definitive host harbours the adult sexually mature worm, whereas intermediate hosts harbour other stages in the life cycle.

effects, or can rupture causing metastatic spread, and become secondarily infected, calcify and/or die.

Eosinophilia is present in less than 25 % of those infected. Diagnosis is by X-ray visualization of cysts with calcified walls, by serological tests, or at operation.

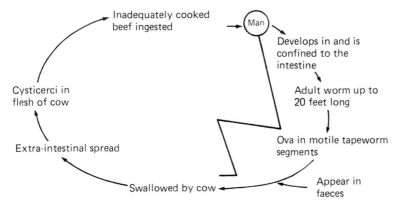

Figure 19   The life cycle of the beef tapeworm

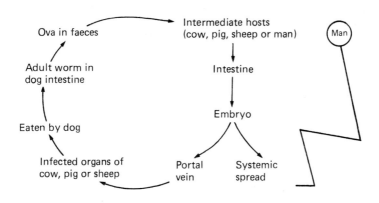

Figure 20   The life cycle of the dog tapeworm

Dwarf tapeworm

Infection is found in tropical, semi-arid areas and usually affects children. Man is the sole host and the worm's life cycle can be completed within a single human host. Diagnosis is by finding eggs in the stool.

Fish tapeworm

Man is a definitive host and there are two sequential intermediate hosts.
Classically this infection is acquired from fish in Scandinavian lakes, but

infection is present elsewhere. Usually patients are asymptomatic but vitamin B12 deficiency may result, possibly producing subacute combined degeneration of the spinal cord.

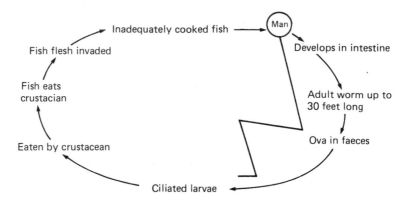

Figure 21   The life cycle of the fish tapeworm

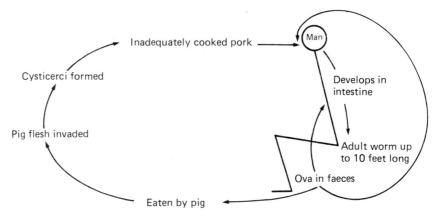

Figure 22   The life cycle of a pig tapeworm. Man is the definitive host (and reservoir) and, in cysticercosis, functions as an intermediate host

Pig tapeworm

In the human, cysticerci (the larval form of the tapeworm) develop about four months after infection, and symptoms are produced depending on their situation. The cysticerci may calcify – a valuable X-ray clue. Fever, headache, urticaria and eosinophilia can occur in the early stages and, usually much later, swellings in muscle become palpable or clinical evidence of cysts becomes apparent (e.g. epileptic fits).

If there is an intestinal tapeworm, diagnosis is by identification of eggs in stool or by examination of an expelled worm. Treatment should not be with drugs that disintegrate tapeworm segments (which would release eggs) because cysticercosis may be initiated.

NEMATODES

Filariasis

These worms have a mosquito to man cycle.

Lymphoreticular filariasis

This occurs in Africa, coastal areas of Asia, Northern South America, the West Indies, Queensland and other areas. The causative worm is usually *Wuchereria bancrofti*, a worm 40–100 mm long, which invades lymphatic tissue causing lymphatic obstruction and fibrosis leading to elephantiasis: when established elephantiasis consists of non-pitting lymphoedema, usually affecting the legs or scrotum. During the acute stage of infection there may be fever, headache and lymphadenopathy. Eosinophilia may be present at any stage.

Diagnosis is by examination of the blood *at night* when microfilaria released by the gravid female adult are circulating. Serological tests are also available.

Treatment is usually with diethylcarbamazine and the appropriate therapy for lymphoedema.

Cutaneous filariasis caused by Loa loa

This is transmitted by Chrysops flies. It is prevalent in certain parts of Africa and causes transient inflamed oedematous swellings mainly on the legs (Calabar swellings). The adult worms may be noted by the patient as they migrate across the eye or beneath the skin. Eosinophilia can be marked. Diagnosis is finding microfilaria in the blood *during the day* or by serological tests including fluorescent antibody testing. Treatment is with diethylcarbamazine.

Cutaneous filariasis caused by Onchocerca volvulus ('River blindness')

This is widely distributed, including some areas of Africa, Mexico, Guatemala and South America. It is transmitted by Simulium flies which are usually found near running water. An initial inflammatory reaction localizes the worms but the female has usually released microfilaria which then migrate causing irritation and fibrosis: clinically there is skin irritation, corneal opacities or skin nodules of various sizes. Eosinophilia is suggestive but diagnosis depends on identification of microfilaria on skin snippings or a positive complement fixation test.

Guinea worm

Transmission is by a crustacean (*Cyclops*) which is accidentally ingested by humans. Subsequently guinea worm larvae penetrate the human intestine and eventually mature into the adult form. Later there is ulceration (usually on the feet where the adult female worm emerges when the limb is exposed to cold water) to liberate larvae infective for *Cyclops*. Treatment is by gentle traction on the worm but niridazole and thiabendazole are also useful prior to traction. Diagnosis is by observing the worms or by X-ray appearance of the calcified dead worms.

Hookworm

Two species of worms can be responsible, *Ancylostoma duodenale* or *Necator americanus*. Hookworm is widely distributed in the tropics where it is a major cause of hypochromic anaemia: an estimated 450 million people are infected

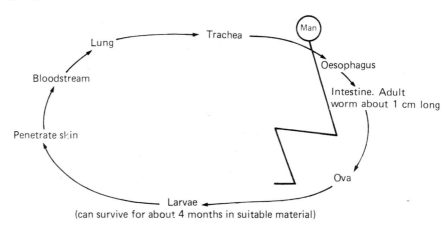

Figure 23   The life cycle of the two human hookworms

Symptoms may occur when the larvae penetrate the skin, usually of the feet, to cause an itchy dermatitis ('Ground itch'). Respiratory symptoms may occur as the larvae pass through the lungs. Mild diarrhoea or vague upper abdominal pain may occur in heavy infections and blood loss may cause anaemia. Eosinophilia may result, especially when the larvae pass through the lungs ('Pulmonary eosinophilia'). If non-human hookworms penetrate the skin the larvae cannot develop further but migrate through the skin until they die – producing a 'persistent ground itch' and an urticarial mobile serpiginous rash (cutaneous larva migrans). Treatment of intestinal infection is with bephenium, thiabendazole or tetrachlorethylene.

Muscle worm

This worm is of worldwide distribution and causes a clinical illness consisting of fever, orbital oedema, myalgia and eosinophilia as a reaction to the migrating larvae of *Trichinella spiralis*. Infection is acquired by ingestion of inadequately cooked pork which contains encysted larvae: in the gut the larvae mature and the adult female worm liberates larvae. These larvae then migrate to striated muscle (including the heart) and to the central nervous system where they may cause fits or encephalitis.

There is usually an eosinophilia and the diagnosis may be confirmed by muscle biopsy. Serological tests are available. The larvae may occasionally be found in the patient's stool.

Roundworm

Symptoms, if any, are caused by obstruction of the intestine or of tubular structures derived therefrom, by allergic reactions as the larvae pass through the lungs (including 'pulmonary eosinophilia'), or by malnutrition.

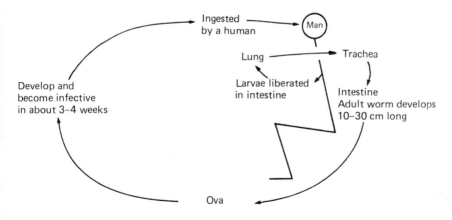

Figure 24   The life cycle of the roundworm

Diagnosis is by identification of the worm or its eggs in the stool and treatment is with piperazine, thiabendazole or bephenium (the latter two being useful as they are also effective against hookworm). If there are multiple infections with worms always treat the roundworm infection first: partial treatment can cause roundworms to get very irritable and troublesome.

Strongyloides

This worm has a wide distribution in tropical areas. Man is the only definitive host.

Symptoms occur when the larvae penetrate and travel rapidly through the skin causing serpiginous, erythematous wheals and oedema. This cutaneous manifestation is cutaneous larva currens and it can occur decades after a patient has left the tropics because the worm can repeatedly

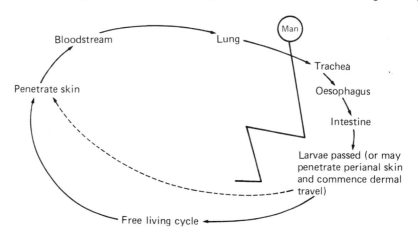

Figure 25   The life cycle of *Strongyloides stercoralis*. This is somewhat similar to hookworm, but hookworm does not have a free living cycle

complete its life cycle in the same host. Symptoms may also occur when larvae pass through the lungs and occasionally mild diarrhoea may result from the intra-intestinal worms. There may be a marked eosinophilia. Diagnosis is by identification of larvae (of which there are two types, A and B, approximately 250 and 600 microns in size respectively) or adult worms in the stool. Treatment is with thiabendazole.

Threadworm

This worm is also known as pinworm or oxyuriasis. The only symptoms are nocturnal anal pruritus or pruritus vulvae (in young girls). Diagnosis is by identification of the worms (the male is about 2–5 mm in size whereas the female is roughly 8–13 mm long) directly in the stool or of the eggs by *the Sellotape strip test* in which tape is applied to a glass slide or a wooden tongue depressor, sticky side out. This is applied early in the morning to the unwashed perianal area. The tape is then transferred, sticky side down, to a clean glass slide. A few drops of xylene are then put onto the slide and microscopic examination will reveal the eggs (55 × 25 microns). Perianal swabs can also be used. Drug treatment is with piperazine adipate, 9 mg

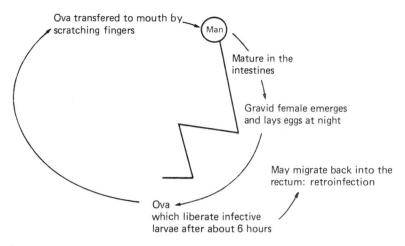

Figure 26   The life cycle of a threadworm

per kg daily for 7 days or viprynium embonate 5 mg per kg as a single dose. Thiabendazole can also be used. As this is commonly a group infection all the family should be treated and frequent changing (and washing) of underclothes, nightwear and bed clothes is indicated. If mothers bring up their children with 'repeated infections' it is important that the infection is confirmed as some mothers develop an 'inner cleanliness' obsession concerning their children: if the infection cannot be confirmed the mother may need vigorous reassurance.

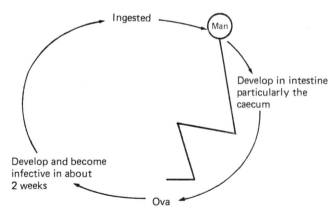

Figure 27   The life cycle of a whipworm

Whipworm

This parasite has a worldwide distribution but is most common in the tropics. If infection is heavy, especially in children, chronic diarrhoea and failure to thrive may result. Mild eosinophilia may be present. Diagnosis is by identification of worms or their eggs in the stool. Treatment is with mebendazole or thiabendazole.

These worms have a complex life cycle with at least one intermediate host, have a gastropod or water snail as the primary host, and have affinity for certain host tissues.

Bilharziasis

There are three main species: *Schistosoma haematobium* which has affinity for the human bladder, *Schistosoma mansoni* and *Schistosoma japonicum*, both of which have an affinity for human intestine and viscera.

Pruritus may be produced when the cercariae penetrate the skin: subsequent pathology is substantially related to the host reaction against the ova produced by the female schistosoma. After infection there may be no symptoms for 5–10 weeks and egg excretion starts about 10–12 weeks after infection.

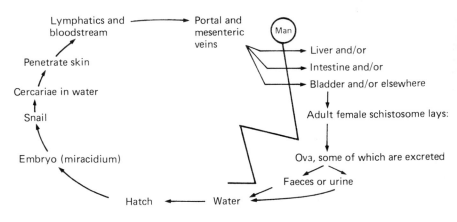

Figure 28   The life cycle of Bilharziasis

The geographical pattern of distribution depends upon the distribution of snails: *S. haematobium* is found in Africa and the Middle East especially Egypt, Greece, Cyprus and Portugal. It usually causes chronic cystitis with fibrosis, metaplasia or malignant change. Clinically there may be terminal haematuria, dysuria, frequency and hydronephrosis. *S. mansoni* is found in Africa, Central and South America, and in the Caribbean area whereas *S. japonicum* is found in the Far East: both may cause acute leading to chronic granulomatous fibrosing inflammation in the colon and rectum possibly leading to ulceration, fistula formation, strictures and predisposition to malignant change. Reactions to ova in the liver cause ('pipestem') fibrosis. A somewhat similar fibrosis may occur in the lungs. Fibrosis, once established, is irreversible unless surgery is possible. Death commonly results from hepatic involvement with portal hypertension and associated illnesses including variceal haemorrhage, or from lung fibrosis leading to cor pulmonale.

Eosinophilia is often present and serological tests are available, but for treatment a diagnosis of active infection has to be substantiated by identification of viable ova in faeces, urine, rectal snippings or tissue biopsy.

Drug treatment is with niridazole or antimony containing compounds (hycanthone, metrifonate or praziquantel).

Other flukes affecting the liver and lung are present in certain areas of the world, mostly in the Orient and Far East, and such infections should be considered in patients from such areas who have liver or lung dysfunction of obscure aetiology. In Britain infection with *Fasciola hepatica* has occurred.

Suggested further reading

Wilcocks, C. and Manson-Bahr, P.E.C. (1974). *Manson's Tropical Diseases. Section 2. Diseases caused by Helminths.* (London: Baillière Tindall)

7
Other infections

Chlamydiae are bacteria-like obligate intracellular parasites. There are two species of chlamydia — A and B.

Chlamydia A

Chlamydia A grows well in columnar epithelium and thus often infects mucosal surfaces of the conjunctivae, cervix, urethra, respiratory tract or gastrointestinal tract. The rectum is particularly vulnerable. Two diseases result.

Trachoma is a keratoconjunctivitis which may lead to corneal scarring. It is a major world cause of blindness and is particularly common in the tropics. A milder illness, known as inclusion conjunctivitis or inclusion blenorrhoea, is probably caused by the same organism which is sometimes known as the TRIC agent (*Trachoma Inclusion Conjunctivitis Agent*).

Lymphogranuloma venereum is a predominantly tropical venereal disease which primarily damages the lymphatic system. In the male there are usually swollen inguinal lymph nodes (buboes) which may suppurate (lymphogranuloma inguinale is another name for this infection). In the female the disease may be occult until complications such as rectal stricture result. Diagnosis is confirmed by demonstrating or cultivating the organism in tissue smears or aspirates, or by serological tests.

Chlamydia B

Chlamydia B causes ornithosis (when derived from any bird) or psittacosis (when derived from psitticine birds including parrots and budgerigars): it is often an occupational disease of bird lovers. Infection is acquired via the respiratory tract. A 'non-typical' pneumonia syndrome results (see Chapter 8). Affected birds may be asymptomatic or have a 'gastroenteritic' or 'chesty' illness.

Diagnosis of chlamydial infection is by isolation of the organism (with an attendant risk of laboratory acquired infection), by microscopic observation of appropriate cytoplasmic inclusions, or by serological tests.

Both species are sensitive to tetracycline or chloramphenicol. Chlamydia A species are usually sensitive to sulphonamides.

INSECTS

Fleas

Infection may occur with human, cat, dog, hedgehog, rabbit, guinea pig or other fleas. There are crops of intensely irritating erythematous macules and papules, possibly with central puncta, weals and excoriations. Papular urticaria may be caused. Treatment is with insecticides.

Lice: Pediculosis humanis

Skin infestation occurs with blood-sucking lice of three varieties: *P. capitis* (head louse), *P. corporis* (body louse) and *Phthirus pubis* (pubic or crab lice). Head and pubic lice attach their eggs (colloquially known as nits) usually, but not always, to their named regions. Lice are transferred directly or on fomites such as clothing in which they may survive for a maximum of about 10 days. Symptoms, if any, are initiated by injection of louse saliva during a blood feed. An itchy red papule results, often with secondary infection consequent to scratching (the lice often defaecate whilst feeding). Hyperpigmentation results from chronic infection.

Treatment with DDT was popular but now other insecticides such as malathion are used but resistance may occur. Retreatment is advisable some 8 days after treatment to ensure that any lice that survived as eggs are eradicated. Heating clothes and other fomites to 50−55°C will kill lice and their eggs within 40 minutes.

Scabies

This skin disease is produced by the mite *Sarcoptes scabiei*. Infection is by close bodily contact, via bedding or via other fomites.

Skin lesions and pruritis are caused by the females which burrow into the stratum corneum of the skin where they deposit faeces and eggs: subsequently the eggs hatch, larvae migrate to the skin surface, mature, and after mating the females start to burrow. There is evidence suggesting that sensitivity plays a major role in pathogenesis because (a) pruritis only starts 4 weeks after an initial infection, (b) a pruritic red papular eruption may appear which bears no relation to the number of mites or their location (Figure 29), and (c) the immunosuppressed develop more florid infections with extensive ulceration and crusting.

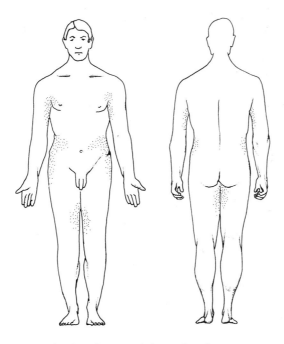

Figure 29   The distribution of the scabies hypersensitivity rash

Norwegian scabies is a florid highly contagious variant of scabies in which there are extensive skin lesions containing large numbers of mites – which may transmit 'standard' scabies to others.

In adults the burrows are usually symmetrical and are almost always present between the fingers and on the wrists: extensor surfaces of the elbows, and the glans penis are other characteristic sites. In children infection can occur virtually anywhere.

Diagnosis is by locating burrows using a magnifying glass and by extracting a mite with a needle.

Treatment is of the patients *and* close contacts: benzyl benzoate or gamma benzene hexachloride are commonly used. After a hot bath, the patient towels down, and the whole body from the neck downwards is painted with either of the two preparations. The patient does not bath again until the next night when the process is repeated. Clothing and bedding should be washed each day. Patients should be given a more detailed printed sheet of instructions to follow.

RICKETTSIAL INFECTIONS

All true rickettsiae except *R. quintana* are unstable outside host cells and thus a vector is usually required for transportation from host to host. Arthropods are common vectors and rickettsiae may well have evolved from arthropod gram negative intestinal bacteria. Depending on the particular vector, there may be a small papule or ulcer (eschar) at the site of the arthropod bite. The rickettsiae have an affinity for vascular endothelium and vascular lesions are characteristic.

The pathogenic rickettsiae are detailed in Figure 30. In general the typhus illnesses consist of abrupt onset fever, chills or rigors, myalgia or arthralgia, headache, anorexia, and a rash which usually occurs about the fifth day of illness: symptoms may persist for variable periods – occasionally up to 4 weeks.

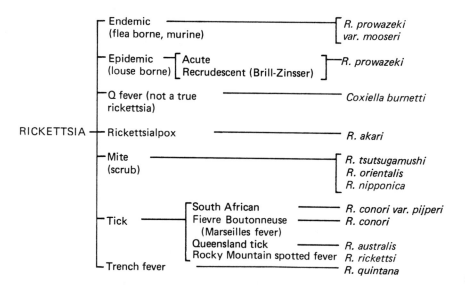

Figure 30   A classification of the common Rickettsial (Typhus) illnesses

Other infections

To confirm a diagnosis of typhus the organism can be isolated but, especially in the case of epidemic typhus, this is not without risk to laboratory staff and is not usually attempted. Direct measurement of typhus antibody in the blood would require typhus antigen for estimation but obtaining this would also be hazardous: fortunately typhus antibodies cross react with certain strains of *Proteus* (OX19, OXK and OX2) and these reactions can be used to detect such antibodies (the Weil–Felix reactions). Differential reactions to the three types of proteus organisms can usefully differentiate between various types of typhus.

Endemic Typhus

Endemic (flea-borne, murine) Typhus is transmitted by a rat flea (*Xenopsylla cheopis*) and is of wide geographical distribution. The mortality rate without treatment is about 5%.

Epidemic Typhus

Epidemic (louse-borne, classical) Typhus is particularly infective because of the ready communicability of the lice and great care is necessary when dealing with and delousing such patients. Clinically, there is high fever, rigors, severe headache, eye suffusion and a stuporose drunken look. (Typhus is derived from a Greek word meaning smoky – referring to the patient's mental haziness.) A rash occurs on the trunk about day 5, later spreading to the periphery. Many years after an acute attack a recrudescence may occur: this is usually a milder illness than the original attack and is known as Brill-Zinsser disease.

Q fever

Q fever is caused by infection with *Coxiella burnetti* (this is not a true rickettsial organism) which can exist extracellularly in the environment for long periods. It is a widespread farming related disease transmitted by dust, droplet aerosols, occasionally by milk, but rarely by ticks. Usually there is an interstitial pneumonia with associated headache, photophobia, sore eyes and limb pains: there is no rash. It is usually only fatal if endocarditis results.

Diagnosis is by measurement of antibody levels to two differing phases of the organism's antigenic constitution: phase II antibodies reflect either acute or chronic illness, whereas phase I antibodies reflect only chronic illness.

Rickettsialpox

Rickettsialpox is a mild illness transmitted by a mouse mite and has occurred in New York City and in the USSR. There is a premonitory red papule (the eschar) followed by a vesicular rash which is often misdiagnosed as chickenpox.

Scrub (mite) Typhus

Scrub (mite) Typhus has a wide geographical distribution, notably South East Asia and the Pacific. An eschar occurs and an illness of 1–4 weeks follows. Meningeal signs may be present and deafness is characteristic.

Tick Typhus

Tick Typhus is of various varieties, and these are usually referred to by the predominant area of their distribution – South African Tick Typhus, for example.

Trench Fever

Trench Fever is a rarely fatal illness transmitted by a tick. Quintana refers to the tendency for this organism to cause bouts of fever every 5 days.

Treatment of all these Rickettsial illnesses is with tetracycline or chloramphenicol. Both of these are bacteriostatic and should be continued for at least 5 days after fever has abated.

PRESUMED INFECTIONS

Cat-scratch disease

A few days after a cat-scratch a papule or pustule develops and within about 2 weeks a slowly progressive regional lymph node enlargement commences: initially the nodes are firm and tender but later may become fluctuant and drain spontaneously with fistula formation. Fever, malaise and headache occur in about one third of patients. Both skin and serological tests are available. Histology of excised nodes reveals a characteristic granulomatous appearance. The causative organism is unknown and thus there is no specific therapy other than surgical excision if required.

Sarcoidosis

Sarcoidosis is a multisystem granulomatous disorder, predominantly of young adults, which occurs in reaction to an agent or agents unknown.

Frequent 'infectious disease' presentations include persistent fever, lymph node enlargement, erythema nodosum, chest X-ray abnormalities, or a febrile arthralgia. In addition to these sarcoidosis may have protean manifestations including central nervous system involvement, hilar lymph node enlargement, hypercalcuria with or without hypercalcaemia, myocardial involvement, polyarthritis, pulmonary infiltrations or skin lesions.

The diagnosis may be suggested if a febrile ill patient has an unexpectedly negative Mantoux test − T lymphocyte mediated immunity is characteristically depressed in sarcoidosis. Histology of nodes and skin lesions may show diagnostic appearances with non-caseating granulomas: liver biopsy is positive in about 70% of sarcoidosis patients even if there is no indication of liver involvement. An injection of intradermal sarcoid antigen (the Kveim-Siltzbach test) produces a typical sarcoid granuloma in patients with the disease − but this response takes at least 4 weeks to become positive.

Acute presentations of sarcoidosis tend to have a good prognosis with a tendency to spontaneous cure with or without the use of anti-inflammatory drugs including steroids. A brisk attack of erythema nodosum with bilateral lymph node enlargement seen on X-ray is virtually diagnostic of sarcoidosis and carries a particularly good prognosis. Insidious onset sarcoidosis is less likely to present as an infectious process and carries a much poorer overall prognosis.

Whipple's disease

This is a chronic diarrhoeal disease with progressive weight loss, in which fever and abdominal pains may occur. Joint pains may precede the diarrhoeal illness. The diagnosis is confirmed by the finding of characteristic small bowel biopsy appearances. Protracted antibacterial therapy, often with penicillin and streptomycin initially followed by tetracycline, results in cure − thus suggesting a bacteria-related aetiology.

Suggested further reading

Schachter, J. (1978). Chlamydial infections. *(N. Engl. J. Med.*, **298**, 428, 490 and 540)

Wilcocks, W. and Manson-Bahr P.E.C. (1974). *Manson's Tropical Diseases. Section 6. Diseases caused by Rickettsiae and Bartonellae.* (London: Baillière Tindall)

8
Respiratory tract infections

CHILDHOOD RESPIRATORY TRACT INFECTIONS (**Figure 31**)

Respiratory tract infections are common in the young as they have no acquired immunity to certain pathogenic agents and their immune systems are not fully mature. In most childhood respiratory tract infections the whole of the respiratory tract is infected, but often symptoms and signs are

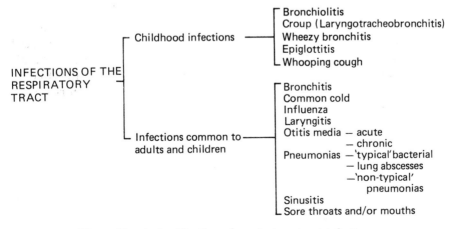

Figure 31 A classification of respiratory tract infections

predominantly of one site. The form the illness takes is often related to the relatively small airways. Recurrent respiratory tract infection in childhood should always raise the possibility of cystic fibrosis (mucoviscidosis).

The possibility of foreign body inhalation or heart failure should not be forgotten in any breathless child. In all recent onset respiratory tract infections in children always look for Koplik's spots – the admission of a child with prodromal measles to a paediatric ward can initiate an epidemic of measles in vulnerable and already ill children.

Bronchiolitis

Although there are several causative agents, bronchiolitis is usually caused by respiratory syncytial virus or parainfluenza viruses. Bronchiolitis often occurs in the winter months and commonly affects infants less than 2 years old, usually 1–6 months old. After a brief upper respiratory tract prodrome there is partial obstruction of terminal branches of the bronchial tree resulting in expiratory wheezing,* intercostal indrawing and *generalized symmetrical* rhonchi on auscultation. Fine inspiratory crepitation may also be audible. Associated hypoxia results in tachypnoea, central cyanosis, tachycardia and restlessness. Often there is reversal of the normal inspiratory-expiratory rhythm, with a pause after inspiration followed by an expiratory grunt. Chest X-ray reveals hyperinflation alone, or occasionally streaky areas of atelectasis. Children with bronchiolitis are often more ill than those with wheezy bronchitis: the clinical picture is unlike asthma – which in any case is unusual in this age group.

Croup (acute laryngotracheobronchitis)

This is characterized by hoarseness, a 'barking' cough, an inspiratory stridor often with forced inspiration and intercostal indrawing: there may be signs related to bronchitis – usually consisting of symmetrical rhonchi perhaps with crepitations. There are many possible causative organisms mostly viral, including parainfluenza type 1, respiratory syncytial virus and influenza. If the child is afebrile and without signs of complications anti-bacterial therapy may be cautiously withheld whilst observing the effect of other therapy. Exhaustion, respiratory obstruction and respiratory failure are the main dangers.

Wheezy bronchitis

This is an ill-defined but clinically recognizable syndrome which often occurs during the course of transient respiratory tract infections. Its relation to asthma is uncertain but it seems likely that infection triggers off

---

*Wheezing = audible rhonchi.

bronchospasm. Clinically there are generalized symmetrical rhonchi without stridor or hoarseness, and often there is a history of previous episodes. A chest X-ray may show hyperinflated but otherwise normal lungs.

The complications of the above three infections are similar – secondary pneumonia (recognized by clinical or X-ray deterioration), atelectasis, otitis media, exhaustion or respiratory failure.

Treatment of the above three syndromes is broadly similar. In mild cases, the importance of adequate hydration should be explained to the parents and arrangements made to provide humidified air (steam kettles etc.). Antispasmodics seem to help wheezy bronchitis but not bronchiolitis. Older children often feel more comfortable if nursed sitting up. If the illness is severe (resting pulse rate above 160/min, marked stridor, severe dyspnoea, cyanosis, shock) or the parents are not able to cope for any reason, the child should be admitted to hospital for more intensive humidified oxygen therapy, attention to the airway and for a chest X-ray to exclude chest complications. Rarely intubation or tracheostomy may be necessary.

Epiglottitis

The incidence is highest in children aged 2–5 years. After an abrupt onset of fever and sore throat, gross swelling of the epiglottis occurs: *Haemophilus influenzae* bacteraemia (the most common causative pathogen) is often present. Often there may be an associated laryngitis or bronchitis. Epiglottitis is a medical (occasionally a surgical) emergency as respiratory obstruction may occur with devastating rapidity. Early epiglottitis may be suspected if a red, swollen, easily visible epiglottis is seen on inspection of a 'sore throat'. Later in the course of illness stridor may occur and, in cases which I have seen, the stridor sounds more proximal than that of croup. If epiglottitis is suspected, one should not attempt to visualize the epiglottis without full anaesthetic facilities as respiratory obstruction may be precipitated. A portable lateral neck X-ray may be useful in differentiating between croup and epiglottitis – an enlarged epiglottis is seen on X-ray in epiglottitis.

Treatment requires *urgent hospital admission:* an adequate airway must be assured and facilities for endotracheal intubation must be kept next to the patient. High dose intravenous ampicillin should be given and some would advocate steroids in addition.

Whooping cough (pertussis)

This is a highly infectious disease with an incubation period of 10–16 days. It can affect *any* age but whoops only occur in young children. The onset is

111

gradual with nasal discharge and cough. The cough becomes more evident over about 2 weeks until the whooping stage occurs. During the whooping stage there are paroxysms of continuous expiratory coughing with production of tenacious sputum; during these paroxysms the child may become cyanosed (or even black) due to anoxia and hypoxic fits may occur. Eventually the paroxysm ends and a vast inspiration causes the characteristic whoop – a prolonged, high pitched 'suction noise'. The whooping stage lasts about 2 weeks and the recovery period thereafter is also about 2 weeks.

Even if whoops are not heard whooping cough may be suspected if there has been contact with whooping cough, if coughing occurs unpredictably in bouts, if there is vomiting at the termination of a coughing bout, and if there is production of sputum – whooping cough is one of the few disorders of children in which sputum is produced rather than swallowed. The finding of a blood lymphocytosis is highly suggestive of whooping cough. Isolation of *B. pertussis* from a pernasal swab confirms the diagnosis. However, such swabs grow *B. pertussis* in less than about 70 % of patients during the whooping stage.

Complications are:

(a) *related to asphyxia*, which may be fatal,
(b) *infective* – bronchopneumonia with atelectasis and otitis media (suspect these if there is a fever in the whooping stage),
(c) *related to pressure changes* – inguinal and umbilical herniae, rectal prolapse, periorbital oedema, subconjunctival and other haemorrhages and (rarely) pneumothorax or mediastinal emphysema,
(d) caused by *central nervous system dysfunction* – hypoxic and 'idiopathic' whooping cough related brain damage may occur.

Infants below the age of six months are the most vulnerable to complications.

Domiciliary management rests upon careful explanation to the parents of the management of a paroxysm and the need for adequate nutrition and adequate fluid intake. Management of a paroxysm consists in positioning the child such that inhalation of vomit is unlikely and so that secretions in the mouth may drain: cough suppressants seem to have little to offer and on theoretical grounds may possibly be harmful. The affected child should be nursed in a quiet, constant temperature environment.

If complications develop or the parents cannot cope for any reason, hospital admission should be advised for constant observation and intensive humidified oxygen therapy if required. Such oxygen therapy can be achieved in an oxygen tent or in infants by using a transparent 'headbox' from which the infant can be removed rapidly when a paroxysm occurs.

The indications for antibacterial therapy are debatable, especially in the whooping stage when the organism may not be cultured. It seems logical to give antibacterial therapy early in the course of the disease, before whooping occurs, in an attempt to prevent deterioration and to reduce infectivity. Once the whooping is established, there is no convincing evidence that antibacterial therapy helps the patient. The prophylactic administration of antibacterial therapy to close contacts is of unproven efficacy but again seems to be logical. If antibacterial therapy is given for whooping cough or for its prevention, erythromycin or co-trimoxazole are appropriate.

RESPIRATORY INFECTIONS COMMON TO ADULTS AND CHILDREN

Bronchitis (acute)

This is most common during winter months and initially consists of substernal discomfort, fever, an initial non-productive cough: later there may be mucopurulent sputum. Diffuse symmetrical rhonchi and occasional crepitations are heard on auscultation of the chest. The chest X-ray is usually normal or shows a vague increase in bronchovascular markings. Especially in patients with chronic bronchitis, an acute attack of bronchitis may merge with bronchopneumonia.

Uncomplicated acute attacks usually have a viral aetiology and aspirin plus a bronchodilator may be helpful. If secondary bacterial infection is suspected antibacterial therapy is indicated. *Haemophilus influenzae* is the bacterium most commonly implicated in acute exacerbations of chronic bronchitis: useful antibacterial drugs include ampicillin (or its derivatives), tetracyclines or co-trimoxazole.

Bronchitis (chronic)

This is said to exist when a chronic recurrent cough with expectoration persists for more than three months of each year. It is essentially a disease of adults which is associated with cigarette smoking and air pollution.

Impairment of ciliary activity and excessive mucus production leads to obstruction of small airways with associated secondary bacterial infection. In an exacerbation there is usually audible wheezing and diffuse rhonchi. Cyanosis is variable: some patients eschew cyanosis and hyperventilate ('pink puffers') whereas others surrender to cyanosis and do not hyperventilate ('blue bloaters').

Patients with chronic bronchitis should avoid rapid temperature changes (such as entering unwarmed bedrooms) which may trigger off bronchospasm. Bronchodilator therapy is of use and antibacterial therapy should be used at the first sign of an exacerbation. Some would recommend prophylactic antibacterial therapy for those at risk. Continuous domiciliary oxygen has its advocates. Regular vaccination against current strains of influenza is essential in this group. Chest physiotherapy (postural drainage, percussion and breathing exercises) is valuable.

Common colds

After an incubation period of 1–4 days there is sneezing, nasal obstruction and profuse rhinorrhoea which is initially mucoid but later mucopurulent. The nasal mucosa is boggy and swollen. Fever is minimal or absent. The common cold syndrome can be caused by a multitude of agents including rhinoviruses (10–25% of colds), coronaviruses, some coxsackie and Echo-viruses, respiratory syncytial virus (usually in adults), adenoviruses and mycoplasma.

Treatment is symptomatic; decongestants containing an antihistamine and atropine-like compounds are useful in drying up secretions. Vitamin C is of unproven efficacy. Antibacterial drugs are not indicated for an uncomplicated attack.

Influenza

After an incubation period of 1–4 days there may be an abrupt onset of fever, malaise, shivering, hacking cough, musculoskeletal pains, sore throat, slight nasal discharge and sneezing. No doubt many attacks are less severe. Influenza should not be confused with the common cold – in which patients are usually afebrile and have a copious nasal discharge.

Classical influenza usually lasts about 4 days and if fever symptoms or signs persist for longer suspect primary influenzal pneumonia or secondary bacterial pneumonia. Secondary bacterial invasion is common with peni-cillin resistant *Staph. aureus* and should be treated with antibacterial drugs.

Diagnosis of influenza is confirmed by isolation of the virus or by sero-logical tests on paired sera.

The treatment of an uncomplicated attack of influenza is symptomatic – aspirin exacerbates perspiration and codeine seems a useful alternative: codeine is also a cough suppressant – which may or may not be a desirable property. Amantidine may also be useful prophylactically, particularly if at risk patients have Parkinson's disease which also improves.

Prevention by vaccination will usually protect the majority of those at risk for about 3–6 months, providing the vaccine includes antigens derived from the current viral strains.

Laryngitis

In children, laryngitis may be the predominant part of the croup syndrome. In adults, infection related laryngitis may present as a seeming-ly distinct entity although the causative organisms (usually viruses) are present elsewhere in the respiratory tract. In adults, there is a barking cough, hoarseness and possibly laryngeal tenderness. Fever and dyspnoea are often minimal or absent.

Treatment includes vocal rest, water saturated air inhalations and oxygen if necessary. If there are other signs suggesting bacterial respiratory tract infection, appropriate antibacterial therapy should be given. Diphtheria and tuberculosis should not be forgotten as possible causes of laryngitis.

Otitis media

Given an intact tympanic membrane acute otitis media is almost invariably secondary to infection derived from the upper respiratory tract; blockage of the eustachian tube or viral invasion of the middle ear may predispose to bacterial infection. Pus, if imprisoned, may force its way into the pneumatized petrous temporal bone or cause perforation of the tympanic membrane. Acute otitis media is most common in children – the eustachian tube seems more vulnerable to obstruction as it is horizontal and because its entrance is surrounded by lymphoid tissue. Clinically there is an abrupt onset of fever, ear ache, conductive deafness and (especially in *Strep. pyogenes* or *Strep. pneumoniae* infection) the tympanic membrane is bulging and fiery red such that the usual bony landmarks may be obscured and the normal light reflex of the tympanic membrane is lost. Otitis media in infants may present in a 'non-focal' fashion with fever, 'unhappiness', failure to feed, meningism, vomiting or diarrhoea.

Haemophilus influenzae is a frequent causative organism in the under fives, and ampicillin or its derivatives are usually the drugs of choice. In older patients, *Strep. pneumoniae*, *Strep. pyogenes* and *Staph. aureus* become more frequent and treatment with the narrower spectrum penicillin is reasonable: erythromycin, a cephalosporin or co-trimoxazole are suitable alternatives in penicillin-allergic patients. Whichever antibiotic is prescribed the need for analgesia should not be forgotten.

Other treatments which may have to be considered in difficult, recurrent or unresponsive cases include myringotomy or adenoidectomy.

Chronic otitis media usually occurs in association with tympanic membrane perforation. Gram negative bacteria including *proteus*, *klebsiella* and *pseudomonas* are common pathogens. Antibacterial therapy (if indicated) should be determined from the results of culture. Meticulous aural toilet, antiseptic agents and later myringoplasty may be required.

Pneumonias

These can be defined as inflammation of the lung with alveolar involvement due to invasion by microorganisms. Although the following classification is not uniformly reliable and is not a substitute for clinical experience, it will help the inexperienced to arrive at sensible therapeutic decisions.

In each case of pneumonia it is essential to attempt to obtain a specimen of sputum and, in hospital practice, to obtain a blood culture prior to initiating treatment.

An immediate Gram stain of sputum may be diagnostically helpful as clusters of gram positive organisms suggest staphylococci, gram negative rods suggest *H. influenzae* unless klebsiella is a possible pathogen, and gram positive cocci in short chains are likely to be *Strep. pneumoniae*.

'TYPICAL' BACTERIAL PNEUMONIAS

Classical lobar pneumonia

Classical lobar pneumonia with diffuse involvement of one or more lobes presents with fever, a dryish cough (perhaps with rusty coloured sputum), dyspnoea and pleuritic chest pain. Herpes febrilis is common. Clinically there are signs of consolidation (chest movement reduced, dullness of the percussion note, bronchial breath sounds, increased vocal resonance and whispering pectriloquy). There is no mediastinal displacement. Later signs of pleural effusion may follow (reduced or absent breath sounds, diminished vocal resonance and a stony dull percussion note). Particularly in children, upper lobe pneumonias may produce delirium or meningism. Chest X-ray reveals diffuse opacity delineated by interlobar fissures. Before initiating antibacterial therapy, sputum and blood cultures should be obtained and a Gram stain of sputum performed. *Strep. pneumoniae* is frequently the causative organism and treatment is with penicillin which should initially be given parenterally (with the exception of certain geographical areas, pneumococci are almost invariably sensitive to penicillin). Oxygen should be given if indicated and analgesia and cough suppression can both be achieved by analgesics such as codeine. If there is a pre-existent chronic respiratory disease, oxygen therapy should be introduced with monitoring of blood gases; some patients may have abandoned their normal carbon dioxide mediated respiratory drive and be dependent on hypoxic drive, and exceeding their normal oxygen concentration by means of oxygen administration will result in hypoventilation and further carbon dioxide retention.

Classical bronchopneumonia

Classical bronchopneumonia is rare in previously fit individuals unless there are predisposing factors. In young children predisposing factors include any lower respiratory tract infection and disorders such as mucoviscidosis; in adults an attack of influenza or pre-existent lung disease may predispose. Bronchopneumonia often starts as an acute bronchitis but fever and discoloured sputum develop. Coarse crepitations may be present in one or more areas of the chest and signs are usually bilateral. There may also be signs of lobar or lobular consolidation.

Haemophilus influenzae is frequently associated with exacerbations of chronic bronchitis. A lobar or more commonly bronchopneumonic picture may result. Ampicillin is usually the drug of first choice, but co-trimoxazole is useful if ampicillin resistance is suspected.

In previously unfit individuals, various other pathogens may be implicated. Diabetes or alcoholism may predispose to *Klebsiella* pneumonia in which there is a rapid progressive necrotizing infection with possible cavitation: a suggestive feature on X-ray is expansion of the affected lobe caused by extensive oedematous inflammation. Drug therapy usually rests on aminoglycosides, cephalosporins or chloramphenicol which may also have a place. Combination therapy is often utilized to prevent rapid emergence of resistant strains.

Pseudomonas aeruginosa tends to cause hospital acquired pneumonias characterized by multiple small abscesses possibly due to vasculitic lesions. Drug therapy is with an appropriate aminoglycoside (usually gentamicin or tobramycin) either alone or in combination with carbenicillin.

Staph. aureus pneumonia usually occurs in the very young, the very old or anyone after an attack of influenza. Drug addicts who unwittingly inject themselves with the organism may present with staphylococcal pneumonia, possibly with an underlying right sided endocarditis. There may be patchy involvement of several pulmonary segments, a predominantly lobar picture, or multiple abscesses perhaps with fluid levels therein – pneumatocoeles. Drug therapy, before the results of sensitivity testing are known, should be with a drug or drugs not inactivated by penicillinase.

Tuberculous pneumonia commonly arises in upper lobes and one should suspect active tuberculosis if there is cavitation and calcification with fluffy surrounding areas on X-ray (lung neoplasms do not often calcify). If a tuberculous abscess ruptures into a bronchus, tuberculous bronchopneumonia results (galloping consumption).

Cavitation in an area of pneumonia should make one suspect staphylococcal pneumonia, tuberculosis, gram negative pneumonias (especially klebsiella), anaerobic pneumonias or necrotizing neoplasms.

Lung abscesses

Severe pneumonic illnesses can cause necrotic areas which develop into lung abscesses. Precipitating causes include influenza, inhalation of food or vomit, foreign body inhalation, underlying carcinoma, septic pulmonary emboli, or right sided endocarditis. The main clinical clue to the presence of lung abscesses is the production of large amounts of foul smelling sputum. On chest X-ray there is cavitation, possibly containing fluid. Complications include empyema formation, metastatic spread of infection, fungal superinfection, or haemorrhage. In about 90% of lung abscesses, anaerobic organisms, such as bacteroides, fusobacteria or anaerobic streptococci, may be isolated; other organisms include *Staph. pyogenes*, klebsiella species, *Strep. pyogenes*, gram negative enteric bacilli, *Myco. tuberculosis*, amoebae, nocardia or fungi. It is essential that adequate specimens of sputum are obtained and are cultured aerobically, anaerobically, for fungi, and for *Myco. tuberculosis*: transtracheal aspiration may be required to prevent contamination with commensal mouth anaerobes.

Conservative treatment is with postural drainage and antibacterial therapy: chloramphenicol is active against most anaerobes whereas penicillin is only active against a few anaerobes. Metronidazole, cefoxitin, clindamycin or lincomycin are also possible drugs for use against anaerobes. If conservative therapy seems unlikely to succeed, surgery should be considered.

'NON-TYPICAL' PNEUMONIAS

By the term 'non-typical' I refer to pneumonias that do not conform to the recognizable standard bacterial pneumonias; pneumonias which fall into this category include those caused by:

adenoviruses,
enteroviruses,
influenza,
Legionnaire's disease,
mycoplasma,
ornithosis, and
Q fever

These pneumonias may be suspected in patients:

(1)   who have no obvious predisposition to standard bacterial pneumonia,
(2)   who are young, previously fit, adults,
(3)   who have failed to respond appropriately to therapy for standard pneumonia. In particular, a persistent protracted irritating cough despite penicillin therapy should suggest ornithosis, mycoplasma or Q fever. Another possibility is whooping cough, which may occur in adults but without the whoop;
(4)   who have marked extrapulmonary symptoms, and
(5)   have sputum that is mucoid.

Specifically suggestive points

Mycoplasma pneumonia, unlike influenza or Q fever, presents with a *gradual onset* of malaise and fever. Headache is a common accompaniment to Q fever, ornithosis and mycoplasma pneumonias. Musculoskeletal aches and pains are common in influenza or ornithosis. In ornithosis there may be diarrhoea, possibly haemoptysis and mental symptoms (such as confusion, delirium and stupor). In ornithosis there may be a history of contact with birds, whereas in Q fever there may be a history of exposure to farm animals.

In all the 'non-typical' pneumonias listed above, the chest X-ray may have patchy areas with uniform or mottled opacity of non-lobar distribution and, particularly in the case of ornithosis or mycoplasma pneumonia, these are often more extensive than physical examination would suggest.

A rash may occur in some adenoviral, enteroviral and mycoplasma pneumonias, whereas there is no rash in influenza or Q fever pneumonias. In adenovirus pneumonia a sore throat and pharyngeal infection may also be evident.

The erythrocyte sedimentation rate may be greatly raised in ornithosis, Legionnaire's disease and mycoplasma pneumonias. In mycoplasma pneumonia cold agglutinins may be present in over 50% of patients and a rapidly performed test* can provide strong circumstantial evidence for mycoplasma infection, although other 'non-typical' pneumonias may occasionally induce cold agglutinins.

Suspicion of these 'non-typical' pneumonias is essential as treatment is often available utilizing drugs that are not first-line drugs for 'typical' bacterial pneumonias.

Tetracycline is active against ornithosis, mycoplasma and Q fever.

Erythromycin is effective against mycoplasma and *Strep. pneumoniae* and is useful if there is doubt as to whether a pneumonia is mycoplasmal or pneumococcal in aetiology. Erythromycin seems to be the drug of choice against Legionnaires' disease.

Chloramphenicol is effective against ornithosis, mycoplasma and Q fever – although many would prefer not to use this drug because of the risk of aplastic anaemia.

Non-typical pneumonias in the immunocompromised may be caused by cytomegalovirus, fungi, nocardia or *Pneumocystis carinii*.

Sinusitis

Sinusitis commonly follows coryza, vasomotor rhinitis, deviation of the nasal septum, polyps, tumours and dental abscesses. There is throbbing pain, tenderness on pressure local to the involved sinus and nasal obstruc-

---

*Add a few drops of blood to the citrate in a commercial prothrombin tube to make a 50/50 mix and place the tube in the freezer section of a refrigerator. Remove the tube after a few minutes. If the tube is tilted and rotated obvious agglutination will be seen on the tube wall if cold agglutinins are present. The agglutination disappears on warming.

tion may be present. Copious purulent nasal discharge occurs if there is rapid drainage of an infected sinus and if the discharge has a foul smell anaerobic infection should be suspected. In maxillary sinusitis the antrum fails to transilluminate. An X-ray may reveal opacification of the sinus, possibly with a fluid level.

Complications include spread of infection with abscess formation, cavernous sinus thrombosis, osteomyelitis of the skull, or meningitis.

Therapy consists of analgesia, water-saturated warm air inhalations, vasoconstrictor agents (to assist ostial opening) and appropriate postural drainage to assist drainage of the affected sinuses. In an acute episode most patients should be given antibacterial therapy. The common pathogens causing acute sinusitis are *Haemophilus influenzae, Strep. pneumoniae* and staphylococci but both mixed infections and anaerobic infections are possible. Initial drug therapy can be with ampicillin or its derivatives, co-trimoxazole or erythromycin. Penicillin is often used successfully although *Haemophilus influenzae* is insensitive. Metronidazole is indicated if anaerobic infection is suspected clinically.

SORE THROATS AND MOUTHS (Table 4)

Table 4   Infection related sore throats and mouths

Viruses
Adenoviruses
Aphthous ulcers
Chickenpox
Cytomegalovirus
Glandular fever
Hand, foot and mouth disease
Herpangina
Herpes simplex
Herpes zoster
Influenza
Measles
Mumps
Rubella

Bacteria
Streptococcal infections
Ludwig's angina
Vincent's angina
Diphtheria

Other causes
Candida
Reiter's syndrome
Stevens–Johnson syndrome
Toxoplasmosis

Bacterial causes

Sore throats are a not uncommon problem in general practice: the results of throat swab culture and blood tests are rarely available rapidly enough to be of immediate diagnostic help, and thus the decision to give an anti-bacterial drug has to be made on the clinical findings. In practice the common problem is to decide which sore throats are streptococcal in aetiology and should be treated with penicillin. In the absence of penicillin hypersensitivity there is rarely an indication to treat sore throats with any antibacterial drug other than penicillin: most penicillin derived drugs have an unnecessary wide spectrum of activity, and ampicillin with its derivatives usually cause rashes if patients have undiagnosed infectious mononucleosis.

Ideally a throat swab from all patients should be taken for bacterial culture into Stuart's transport medium. If streptococci are grown treatment should be continued for a total of 10 days, but if no streptococci are grown then treatment can be discontinued. A positive culture for streptococci from a 'quiet' throat indicates a carrier state which under normal circumstances requires no therapy.

Lancefield group A β-haemolytic streptococci (Strep. pyogenes)

These may cause pharyngitis, tonsillitis or quinsy (peritonsillar abscess) with possible sequelae such as rheumatic fever or glomerulonephritis. In a classical streptococcal sore throat there is an abrupt onset illness with fever and headache: earache is typical but nasal stuffiness and discharge are not prominent. Dysphagia is usually caused by lancinating pain rather than by obstruction. On examination there is redness and congestion of the throat, the tonsils are enlarged with 'cheesy' exudates emanating from the tonsillar crypts. *Such exudates do not spread beyond the tonsils.* Particularly in young children exudates may not be present. Cervical lymph node enlargement is usually noted after the onset of symptoms and signs local to the throat. Scarlet fever is usually caused by group A β-haemolytic streptococcal tonsillitis associated with a white-then-red 'strawberry' tongue and the characteristic rash. A unilateral quinsy causes midline shift and gross swelling of the pharyngeal structures in addition to the symptoms and signs of streptococcal pharyngitis.

Which sore throats should be treated as if they were streptococcal in aetiology? Certainly those in which the appearances suggest streptococcal infection (typical streptococcal exudates can occur in viral infections but should be presumed to be streptococcal pending throat swab results). Patients with streptococcal complications should be treated, including patients with a quinsy (most resolve with intramuscular penicillin therapy without the need for incision), retropharyngeal abscess, otitis media or scarlet fever. Patients who have defective host defences or a previous attack of rheumatic fever or chorea should be treated and, finally, patients whose occupation brings them into close contact with susceptibles – nurses and doctors for example – should be started on a course of penicillin, and should stay off work pending the results of the throat swab.

Treatment of streptococcal sore throats is with penicillin G (intramuscularly) or penicillin V (orally) depending upon the severity of the infection. In general practice triple preparations of penicillin which contain a short, medium and long acting penicillin are a useful one injection treatment as patients often discontinue oral therapy once the symptoms have subsided (with attendant risk of relapse). Erythromycin is a useful alternative to penicillin in the penicillin allergic patient.

Ludwig's angina (submandibular cellulitis)

This is commonly streptococcal in aetiology but occasionally is caused by anaerobes. The main danger is that of respiratory obstruction. Treatment is usually with penicillin, but some would also use steroids if respiratory obstruction was impending. Passage of a naso-laryngeal tube may also 'buy time'.

Vincent's angina

Vincent's angina is caused by a double infection with *Fusobacterium fusiforme* and *Borrelia vincenti* resulting in an acute gingivostomatitis, often with ulceration and a grey pseudomembrane with bleeding on attempted removal. It usually occurs in debilitated or leukaemic patients. Treatment is with antiseptic mouthwashes, oral hygiene, penicillin or metronidazole. Tetracyclines are useful if the patient is not immunocompromised.

Diphtheria

Although uncommon if all the population is immunized, it is a diagnosis not to be missed. Pyrexia is usually low grade or absent and in classical cases the characteristic membrane is sharply demarcated with a wrinkled edge, not confined to the tonsils, thick, homogeneous, firmly adherent and later surrounded by a narrow zone of inflammation. In mild tonsillar diphtheria there may be only a small spot of yellowish white membrane with a wrinkled edge: the colour is rarely as pure white as an early infectious mononucleosis exudate may be. In pharyngeal diphtheria the membrane spreads away from the tonsils. This membrane usually has a thick edge and its colour changes rapidly to a green and black hue. However, the membrane may be only a thin, slimy film which is easily missed on a cursory examination. Ulceration is not a feature and bleeding occurs on attempted removal of the membrane. There may be an associated non-painful 'bull-neck' with regional adenitis and the sufferer may be generally floppy and ill: sequelae result from either the occurrence of unpredictable respiratory obstruction due to membrane extension or from the effects of the powerful exotoxin on the heart or the nervous system.

Treatment is by urgent administration of antitoxin *on suspicion* of the diagnosis, protection of the airway, and by penicillin to eliminate the organism. (Erythromycin is an alternative in the penicillin allergic and is also used to treat diphtheria carrier states.)

Other bacteria such as *Haemophilus influenzae* or *Strep. pneumoniae* may cause sore throats but as both may be isolated from normal throats their pathological significance is often uncertain. Group C and Group G *β*-haemolytic streptococci may be responsible for pyogenic sore throats.

Viral sore throats and mouths

Viral infections cause the majority of sore throats and mouths. On occasion viral infections may be clinically indistinguishable from streptococcal infections and indeed may predispose to secondary bacterial infections. In viral sore throats, the white cell count is commonly normal or low and the erythrocyte sedimentation rate is often normal.

Treatment of viral sore throats or mouths is usually symptomatic: hydrocortisone pellets are useful in aphthous ulceration, and local anaesthetics are often useful for painful lesions around the gums despite the risk of sensitivity developing. I find whiskey has a soothing effect on local lesions and allays despair if subsequently swallowed. Antiseptic mouth washes and gargles may be symptomatically helpful although their action can be only superficial. Aspirin gargles are often appreciated.

The above therapies can help to assuage the constant demand for 'an antibiotic please, doctor.'

Adenoviruses

These cause varied clinical pictures depending on the particular adenovirus involved: one characteristic syndrome comprises fever, pharyngitis and conjunctivitis (pharyngoconjunctival fever).

Aphthous ulcers

These are irritating, painful, small (circa 0.5 cm in diameter) ulcers or vesicles which are presumed to be caused by viruses. Individual ulcers begin as shallow erosions with a yellowish raised border surrounded by a narrow, bright red zone. They may be related to mental stress, physical stress or underlying organic disease. As an isolated finding, they usually have no serious significance. Recurrent attacks are common.

Chickenpox

Oral poxes occur in association with the characteristic skin rash.

Cytomegalovirus

A monospot-negative glandular fever syndrome may result with a (relatively uncommon) exudative tonsillitis.

Infectious mononucleosis

In the classical anginose form the oropharynx may be reddened and the tonsils enlarged. Initially the tonsillar appearances are non-specific. Later the characteristic exudate formation may develop: initially, this is usually strikingly white and is confined to the enlarged tonsils, is superficial and can be pushed off easily to leave a red, but non-bleeding area beneath. Palatal petechiae are characteristic of infectious mononucleosis but not diagnostic. If cervical lymph node enlargement occurs before the onset of a sore throat, this favours infective mononucleosis rather than streptococcal infection. In infectious mononucleosis the throat usually is less painful than an uncomplicated streptococcal sore throat and dysphagia is more often caused by obstruction than by pain.

Hand, foot and mouth disease

This is commonly caused by coxsackie A16 virus and consists of slightly painful bright red macules or vesicles surrounded by a red ring about 3–8 mm across. Lesions are present on the feet, hands and in the mouth, particularly on the buccal mucosa and palate: unlike *Herpes simplex* infection there are usually no lesions on the outside of the lips or face.

Herpangina

This is usually caused by a coxsackie A virus and results in an abrupt onset sore throat and dysphagia. The fauces and pharynx are red and distinct greyish papules 1–2 mm in diameter or shallow ulcers up to 5 mm in diameter are surrounded by a red halo. These lesions are present almost exclusively in the back of the mouth, a finding unusual in *Herpes simplex* infection.

Herpes simplex

After a primary infection in children, an acute gingivostomatitis may result with greyish yellow ulcers, often serpiginous, on an inflamed base and predominantly affecting the front of the mouth. Outside the mouth, there are clusters of vesicles which rapidly crust. The tongue is often coated and there may be an associated cervical lymph node enlargement and excessive salivation with secondary implantation of infection due to dribbling may occur.

Recurrent *Herpes simplex* usually involves the lips and systemic symptoms are rare.

Herpes zoster

Herpes zoster, if of maxillary or mandibular distribution, may present as a unilateral oral pain which is rapidly followed by the classical shingles eruption.

Influenza

Sore throat is not usually a major complaint compared with the fever, chills, malaise, headache or myalgia typical of this illness.

Measles

Children especially may complain of a sore throat as part of the prodrome. There will be an associated conjunctivitis and coryza and Koplik's spots should be visible at this stage: these resemble grains of salt scattered on the reddened buccal mucosa.

Mumps

This illness may cause a mild sore throat due to decreased salivation: parotitis may be evident or subsequently develop and the affected salivary duct orifices are often prominent and reddened.

Other causes of sore throats and mouths

Behçets syndrome

This syndrome comprises episodes of oral and genital ulceration of vasculitic aetiology.

Candida (Thrush)

Candida causes creamy white areas which cover inflamed mucous membranes. Common predisposing causes include antibacterial therapy, diabetes mellitus, immune deficiencies, the contraceptive pill and steroid therapy. Treatment is with either nystatin or amphotericin B.

Reiter's syndrome

Reiter's syndrome is strictly recognized by the triad of arthritis, urethritis and conjunctivitis but some patients also have mucocutaneous manifestations which may include a sore mouth.

Stevens–Johnson syndrome

Usually there is inflammation and ulceration of the mouth and mucous membranes (including those of the conjunctivae and genital tract) in association with erythema multiforme. It is a reaction pattern to a variety of stimuli. Steroids may be useful therapy if systemic toxicity dictates or spontaneous resolution is slow.

Toxoplasmosis

A monospot-negative glandular fever syndrome may occur in which pharyngitis is not a common symptom.

Suggested further reading

Hoeprich, P.D. (1977). *Infectious Diseases, Sections 4, 5 and 6.* (London: Harper and Row)

9
Jaundice

Jaundice can be caused by four mechanisms (Figure 32).

(1) *Haemolysis*. Breakdown of haemoglobin and other similar pigments produces *unconjugated* bilirubin: if the ability of the liver to conjugate unconjugated bilirubin is exceeded jaundice results. As unconjugated bilirubin is insoluble in water the excess bilirubin is not excreted into the urine.

(2) *Decreased uptake or conjugation of unconjugated bilirubin by the liver*. This causes an *unconjugated* hyperbilirubinaemia.

(3) *Diffuse cholestasis*. By this I refer to the failure of bile flow or decreased secretion of conjugated bilirubin into the biliary tract *without the presence of a focal space-occupying lesion*. There is a *conjugated* hyperbilirubinaemia. Conjugated bilirubin is water soluble and the excess in the blood passes into the urine (bilirubin-uria). The stool is pale due to lack of bile pigments in the gut.

(4) *Mechanical obstruction of bile flow*. By this I refer to the presence of a focal space-occupying lesion affecting the biliary tract (such as impacted gallstones or a neoplasm) which causes obstruction to the

127

bile flow. This results in a *conjugated* hyperbilirubinaemia with bilirubinuria and a pale stool. If there is a persisting complete obstruction no bile will reach the gut, no urobilinogen will be formed, and urobilinogen will be persistently absent from the urine.

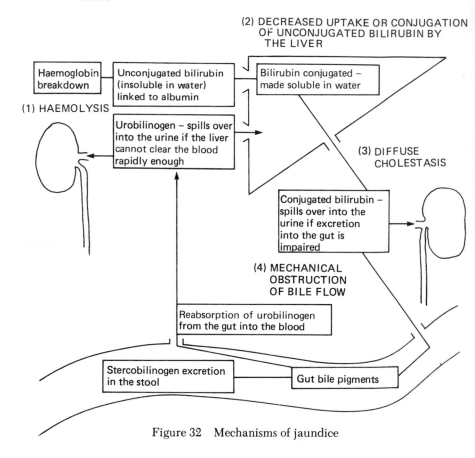

Figure 32   Mechanisms of jaundice

In any patient with jaundice one or more of the mechanisms outlined above may be operating. An accurate working diagnosis can often be made from the history, examination of the patient, urine testing and a few relevant blood tests.

CLINICAL IDENTIFICATION OF THE MECHANISMS OF JAUNDICE

(1)   *Haemolytic jaundice.* There may be a family history of haemolytic disease or a history of ingestion of haemolysis inducing drugs. Haemolytic jaundice is usually mild and 'delicately yellow'. The

liver is not usually tender and there may be splenomegaly. There will be no bile in the urine (an acholuric jaundice) but there will be an excess of urobilinogen in the urine.

(2) *Jaundice due to decreased uptake or conjugation of unconjugated bilirubin by the liver.* There may be a history of transitory mild jaundice with previous infections of a non-hepatitic nature. Apart from mild jaundice the clinical examination is normal and there is no bile in the urine. Some drugs, notably chloramphenicol and progestational steroids, can cause jaundice by this mechanism.

(3) *Jaundice due to diffuse cholestasis.* The clinical diagnosis requires recognition of the various disease patterns which may be responsible (see later). Conjugated hyperbilirubinaemia unlike unconjugated hyperbilirubinaemia, may give rise to pruritis or bradycardia. In an acute viral hepatitis causing diffuse cholestasis, the liver is often diffusely enlarged and tender.

(4) *Jaundice due to mechanical obstruction of bile flow.* Obstructive jaundice has an intense greenish hue – unlike the yellow colour of

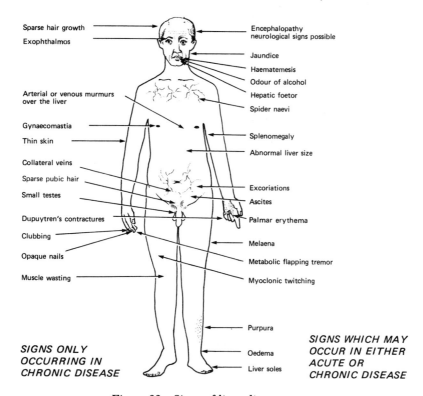

Figure 33   Signs of liver disease

129

haemolytic jaundice. A history of previous biliary tract surgery provides circumstantial evidence for biliary stricture or gallstone impaction. In gallstone impaction there may be a history of biliary colic which may have *preceded* the passage of dark urine. An irregular liver edge or surface points towards mechanical obstruction probably caused by malignancy or cirrhotic nodule formation (marked hepatic regeneration after an episode of hepatic necrosis may cause an irregular liver edge or surface – but this is uncommon). *Focal* liver tenderness in a diffusely enlarged but generally non-tender liver also suggests mechanical obstruction, rather than a diffuse cholestasis: if there is focal tenderness in the gallbladder area (at the junction of the rectus sheath and the rib cage) biliary system pathology is likely. Cachexia suggests chronic liver disease or underlying malignancy. With the exception of palmar erythema and spider naevi, signs of chronic liver disease (Figure 33) are not found in recent onset viral cholestasis. Splenomegaly is not usually an early feature of mechanical biliary obstruction.

FURTHER INVESTIGATIONS OF THE MECHANISM OF JAUNDICE

(1) *Haemolysis*

If haemolysis is significant there will be anaemia with signs of increased red cell production (reticulocytosis and a hyperactive bone marrow), and the haemoglobin binding protein (haptoglobin) will be depleted due to excessive utilization: if there is gross intravascular haemolysis haemoglobinuria may be found.

Examination of a stained blood film may reveal signs of congenital erythrocyte abnormality or evidence of various infections which may cause haemolysis (malaria for example).

Other tests which may be indicated include haemoglobin electrophoresis, glucose-6-phosphate deficiency assay, osmotic fragility tests, Coombs test, and tests for cold agglutinins.

(2) *Decreased uptake or conjugation of unconjugated bilirubin by the liver*

Usually mild hyperbilirubinaemia is the only significant abnormality. Liver function tests are otherwise normal.

(3/4) *Differentiation between jaundice due to diffuse cholestasis or mechanical obstruction*

In practice this differentiation is of paramount importance because surgery in diffuse cholestasis may precipitate hepatic failure, whereas the appropriate surgery may be essential to relieve a mechanical obstruction. This differentiation is assisted by relatively simple blood tests.

Diagnostic clues from blood tests (Table 5)

Haemoglobin level

The haemoglobin level is usually normal in recent onset diffuse cholestasis caused by viral hepatitis, unless the causative infection also causes haemolysis or a bleeding tendency.

Table 5 Suggested initial blood tests in a jaundiced patient. If hepatitis B is a possibility great care should be used in taking blood, and the specimens should be packaged and labelled appropriately (Chapter 15)

Haemoglobin	
White cell count + differential	Consider the need for these if a patient is likely to have
Erythrocyte sedimentation rate	uncomplicated hepatitis B
Heterophil antibody test	

"Liver function tests"
  HBsAg
  Total bilirubin
  (congugated + uncongugated)
  Aspartate transaminase
  Alkaline phosphatase
  Prothrombin time

A stained blood film examination

A pancytopenia suggests hypersplenism which is usually associated with chronic liver disease or bone marrow dysfunction. Very rarely hepatitis A causes an aplastic anaemia. The atypical mononuclear cells of infectious mononucleosis (less commonly cytomegalovirus infection or toxoplasmosis) may be seen.

The erythrocyte sedimentation rate (ESR)

The ESR is usually normal or only slightly raised in hepatitis A or B – the inflamed liver being unable to manufacture sufficient of the relevant factors to elevate the ESR. A grossly raised ESR is distinctly unusual in an uncomplicated episode of viral hepatitis and rather suggests underlying malignancy, certain immune mediated diseases (including systemic lupus erythematosus) or active chronic hepatitis.

A leukocytosis

A leukocytosis (more than 10×10^9 cells per litre) suggests bacterial infection, acute alcoholic hepatitis or leptospirosis. A leukocytosis is unusual in viral infections causing jaundice, apart from fulminant hepatitis and infectious mononucleosis. The coincidence of leukocytosis, jaundice, and renal failure points towards leptospirosis.

A neutropenia

A neutropenia (less than 2.0×10^9 cells per litre) may be found in hepatitis A or B.

A lymphocytosis

A lymphocytosis (more than 4.0×10^9 cells per litre) in the presence of jaundice suggests viral infections including hepatitis A or B, infectious mononucleosis, toxoplasmosis or cytomegalovirus infection. A lymphocytosis speaks against mechanical obstruction. Bacterial illnesses which occasionally cause jaundice with an associated lymphocytosis include typhoid fever, brucellosis, tuberculosis or syphilis.

An eosinophilia

An eosinphilia (more than 0.4×10^9 cells per litre) in association with jaundice suggests a drug reaction or tropical parasite induced liver disease.

A positive monospot test

This test (sometimes referred to as the Paul Bunnell test) confirms infectious mononucleosis – false positives are very rare.

Urea and electrolytes

A raised urea level should suggest leptospirosis. A raised urea level is distinctly unusual in uncomplicated hepatitis A or B as the liver cannot produce the normal quantity of urea, and the prodromal anorexia no doubt also reduces the protein load on the liver.

Bilirubin

In viral hepatitis the swollen liver causes compression of the bile canaliculi which interferes with bile flow: the resulting hyperbilirubinaemia is *predominantly* conjugated (the inflamed liver also has difficulty in dealing with its normal load of unconjugated bilirubin). In practice the fractionation of bilirubin into conjugated and unconjugated elements is seldom of practical help in differentiating jaundice of diffuse cholestasis from that of mechanical obstruction. Certain rare disorders (Dubin Johnson and Roter syndromes) can affect the excretion of conjugated bilirubin into the biliary tract.

Aspartate transaminase (AST)

This enzyme is liberated from damaged bodily tissue, including skeletal and cardiac muscle damage and liver cell damage. Large AST elevations (above 400 IU per litre) usually reflects widespread hepatocellular damage which may be of viral, toxic, drug or ischaemic aetiology. In a jaundiced patient the finding of an elevated AST is useful for the diagnosis of hepatitis and for following its course: the AST usually exceeds 200 IU per litre at some stage in the course of a viral hepatitis. If a patient is jaundiced, has bile in the urine and the AST is normal or only minimally raised it is likely that there is a mechanical obstruction of the biliary tract. A simultaneously raised alkaline phosphatase level would make this conclusion almost certain, although functional obstruction following an attack of hepatitis (posthepatitic cholestasis) is a possible but less likely alternative. Precipitous falls in the AST during the course of a viral hepatitis are an ominous sign, often preceding clinical manifestations of hepatic failure.

Alkaline phosphatase

Alkaline phosphatase (normally less than 105 IU per litre) is produced by osteoblastic activity, irritated biliary epithelium, the intestine and the placenta. If there is concern that high levels may be caused by osteoblastic activity in bone rather than by liver pathology, isoenzymes (including leucine aminopeptidase or 5-nucleotidase) which are not produced by bone can be measured. Very high alkaline phosphatase values favour mechanical obstruction, whereas low values usually exclude this diagnosis. In uncomplicated viral hepatitis the alkaline phosphatase rarely exceeds 2.5 times normal. The alkaline phophatase may also be raised in primary biliary cirrhosis, in intrahepatic space-occupying lesions, occasionally in prolonged post-hepatic cholestasis and occasionally in drug induced diffuse cholestasis.

Prothrombin time

This is prolonged if the liver cannot synthesize prothrombin from vitamin K, or if dietary vitamin K does not reach the liver because of malabsorption from the gut. If there is mechanical biliary tract obstruction a prolonged prothrombin time will rapidly return to normal with parenteral vitamin K administration, as the hepatocellular function is usually intact. In the presence of diffuse hepatocellular dysfunction parenteral vitamin K will only slowly return a prolonged prothrombin time to normal. As most episodes of viral hepatitis are of relatively short duration the prothrombin time is usually normal; a markedly prolonged prothrombin time would suggest impending liver failure.

Serum proteins

Albumin is produced in the liver and a low albumin level may occur in *chronic* liver disease: in an acute hepatitis the albumin level does not have time to fall before liver function recovers (the half-life of albumin is about 3 weeks). An increase in the globulins is a reactive feature usually not found in the relatively brief duration hepatitis A or B; increased globulins are suggestive of chronic liver disease.

The Australia antigen

The presence of the surface antigen of hepatitis B virus (HBs Ag) in a jaundiced patient usually indicates acute hepatitis B. However some patients with hepatitis B may have cleared the HBs Ag prior to the development of jaundice: in such patients one can only make the diagnosis of hepatitis B by demonstrating a rising titre of *antibody* to HBs Ag. One must also beware of HBs Ag carriers who develop jaundice for reasons other than acute hepatitis B.

Serological tests for hepatitis A antibodies are now available. If antibodies are detected this confirms past or present A infection: hepatitis A specific IgM is raised during a current infection.

The mitochondrial fluorescent antibody test. This is positive in most patients with primary biliary cirrhosis, is rarely positive in viral hepatitis, and is usually negative in uncomplicated biliary tract obstruction.

Antinuclear factor and lupus erythematosus cell preparation

If present these indicate immune reactions not usually associated with acute viral hepatitis.

Blood cultures

These should be sterile in a viral hepatitis. They may be positive in leptospirosis, but certain leptospires cannot be cultured and have to be diagnosed by serological tests.

Other tests

These may include serum copper and copper binding protein (caeruloplasmin) to exclude Wilson's disease, protein electrophoresis to identify antitrypsin deficiency, and α-fetoprotein estimation if hepatoma is suspected.

Other tests in the diagnosis of jaundice of uncertain aetiology

Patients in whom the diagnosis is obscure after the above liver function tests have been performed are usually too deeply jaundiced for cholecystography or non-operative cholangiography to yield useful results. A *plain X-ray* of the abdomen may reveal gallstones (about 20% are radioopaque) which may be relevant to the jaundice or which may be only a coincidental finding. Routine *liver biopsy* has no place in the investigation of straightforward viral hepatitis and is only indicated if the diagnosis remains uncertain or if it is suspected that hepatitis B is progressing to active chronic hepatitis. Abdominal *ultrasound examination*, radioactive *isotope scanning* of the liver, *endoscopic canulation* of the ampulla of Vater, percutaneous *cholangiography*, or *peritoneoscopy* may reveal space-occupying lesions incompatible with a diagnosis of viral hepatitis.

CLINICAL SYNDROMES

Infections that may cause haemolytic jaundice

Septicaemia

Septicaemia with any organism may cause red cell disruption sufficient to cause jaundice.

Clostridium perfringens

Clostridium perfringens sepsis, including gas gangrene, is often associated with systemic haemolysis particularly if septicaemia supervenes.

Mycoplasma infection

Mycoplasma infection with associated cold agglutinins may cause haemolysis. Do not let the patient become chilled!

Certain infections may initiate an episode of haemolysis in patients with glucose-6-phosphate deficiency or sickle cell trait or disease.

Syphilis

Syphilis may cause an antibody mediated haemolysis.

INFECTIONS ASSOCIATED WITH DIFFUSE CHOLESTASIS

Hepatitis A and B

Hepatitis A is usually a disease of young people. There may be a history of contact with a jaundiced person, travel abroad, or shellfish ingestion

15–40 days previously. Hepatitis B patients can be of any age: predisposing factors include exposure to blood or blood related products, 'medical' injections, dubious sexual contacts, 'main-line' or subcutaneous drug abuse, or tattooing 40–180 days previously. Both hepatitis A and B may be preceded by a febrile prodrome, a period with dark urine, pale stool, nausea, vomiting and generalized aches and pains. In both hepatitis A and B the prodromal malaise and fever usually remit with the onset of jaundice. A persisting fever in the face of jaundice may be caused by other infective causes of jaundice (for example infectious mononucleosis or cytomegalo-virus hepatitis), by drug reactions, by underlying malignancy, or by acute or subacute hepatitic necrosis. A diagnostically confusing occurrence is a vital hepatitis-like prodrome before the onset of methyldopa or chlorpro-mazine induced hepatitis.

In diffuse hepatitis the liver is usually both diffusely enlarged and tender. If there is associated abdominal pain the passage of dark urine often precedes the pain, whereas the reverse may occur as a gallstone passes down the biliary tract.

Jaundice due to hepatitis A or B usually persists for 1–2 weeks, occasionally longer.

Non-A, non-B hepatitis

There is probably more than one agent which can cause this hepatitis. Non-A, non-B hepatitis may account for up to 90% of all cases of post-transfusion hepatitis as well as many sporadic cases. There is a tendency to long lasting viraemia and progression to chronic hepatitis. The average incubation period varies between 5 and 8 weeks.

Infectious mononucleosis

A mild cholestatic jaundice occurs in about 5–10% of patients with infectious mononucleosis: suggestive lymph node enlargement or tonsillar appearances may be present. A palpable spleen occurs in about 50% of patients with infectious mononucleosis (a palpable spleen occurs in about 20% of patients with hepatitis A or B).

Cytomegalovirus hepatitis

This may present with an infectious mononucleosis-like disease: spleno-megaly, hepatomegaly and atypical lymphocytes in the blood are commonly associated, but sore throat and cervical lymph node enlarge-ment are usually not a feature. Cytomegalovirus infection with hepatitis may occur sporadically, if there is an underlying disease, or 2–4 weeks after a blood transfusion: there is a febrile illness lasting 2–3 weeks with a hepatitis of variable degree with or without jaundice. Occasionally there is an associated maculopapular rash.

Toxoplasmosis

Symptomatic infections include mild febrile illnesses with lymph node enlargement, malaise, muscle pains and slightly altered liver function. Acute fulminating disease may occur, especially in the immunologically compromised, consisting of high fever, a rash and hepatitis. Although toxoplasmosis hepatitis is rare it is treatable with sulphonamides and pyrimethamine or possibly spiramycin.

Q fever

This may rarely cause a granulomatous hepatitis in which jaundice may be a feature.

Yellow fever

An abrupt onset of illness comprising fever, chills, headache, backache, prostration, followed by jaundice and vomiting along with a bleeding tendency and gross albuminuria 3–6 days after return from central Africa, mid or South America is suggestive of this disease.

Drug reactions

Drug reactions are a common non-infective cause of diffuse cholestasis – see Table 6.

Table 6   The main drugs that may cause jaundice

Haemolytic	'Hepatitic'	Cholestatic
Nitrofurantoin	Carbon tetrachloride	Phenothiazines
Many drugs in G6PD	Erythromycin esteolate	Erythromycin esteolate
deficient patients	Paracetamol	Some steroid preparations
including primaquine,	Monoamine oxidase	including the contraceptive
aspirin, sulphonamides	inhibitors	pill and methyltestosterone
	PAS	Chlorpropamide
	Sulphonamides	
	Methyldopa	
	Phenindione	
	Halothane	

Liver failure

A brief illness with jaundice and impaired mental function, a metabolic flapping tremor, or a bleeding tendency indicates diffuse hepatic failure which is almost always caused by fulminant viral hepatitis or by drug toxicity. It is possible to die from fulminant hepatitis before jaundice has developed.

TREATMENT OF HEPATITIS

Treatment is essentially symptomatic and supportive: there is no useful drug treatment for uncomplicated viral hepatitis. Corticosteroids may well achieve a 'whitewash' but they have not been shown to be of use in the routine management of hepatitis or in the management of fulminant hepatitis.

Bed rest seems sensible whilst there is a continuing hepatitis, although the benefit may be marginal for jaundiced patients who are otherwise well.

Isolation may be indicated, although patients with hepatitis A have passed the period of maximum infectivity by the time jaundice is evident. Undiagnosed patients with anicteric hepatitis A are probably of more significance in the transmission of infection. Patients with hepatitis B should be made aware of, but not terrified by, the potential infectivity of all their bodily fluids. Patients with viral hepatitis should probably have their own cutlery, toilet facilities and should not share toothbrushes, razors and such like.

PROGNOSIS OF HEPATITIS

Hepatitis A, infectious mononucleosis hepatitis, and yellow fever do not progress to chronic liver disease: if life threatening complications do not arise during the acute stage the patients can be reassured of ultimate recovery even though liver function tests may take some time to return to normal.

Hepatitis B usually resolves and the virus is cleared from the blood shortly after clinical recovery. However, progressive disease may occur especially if the virus is not cleared from the blood. Active chronic hepatitis, cirrhosis, hepatoma, or other immune mediated disease may subsequently develop.

Suggested further reading

Sherlock, S., and Summerfield, J.A. (1979). *A Colour Atlas of Liver Diseases*. (Oxford: Wolfe Medical Publications Ltd)

Sherlock, S. (1975). *Diseases of the Liver and Biliary System*. (Oxford: Blackwell)

10
Persistent pyrexias of unknown origin

Rather than discussing classical 'pyrexia of unknown origin' (a fever persisting for 2–3 weeks in the absence of an obvious cause), I shall deal with febrile conditions persisting for longer than *several days* in which the clinical history and examination have suggested no obvious diagnosis or diagnoses: such fevers commonly provide diagnostic and therapeutic problems.

All persisting fevers (defined as above 37 °C) except minor elevations in the afternoon and evening should be viewed with suspicion: normally the body temperature is lowest in the early morning and a fever at that time is likely to be significant. Night sweats tend to accompany febrile illnesses as the body attempts to attain this low morning temperature by means of fluid evaporation.

Fever occurs in nearly all significant invasive infections, after extensive trauma, in some collagen or immune mediated diseases, some metabolic diseases, and in association with some neoplasms and vascular incidents. Some blood diseases result in fever with or without the presence of complicating infection.

The pattern of fever may be suggestive of certain diseases but is hardly ever diagnostic and on occasion may even be positively misleading: much the same comment applies to the relative bradycardia which sometimes occurs in some infections, notably typhoid (normally the pulse rate increases by about 18 beats for every degree centigrade rise in temperature).

A *continued pyrexia* is a continuously elevated temperature usually fluctuating by less than 1 °C.

An *intermittent pyrexia* consists of temperature peaks with returns to normal.

A *remittent pyrexia* consists of temperature elevation for all or most of the day with a difference between the maximum and minimum of 1 °C or more.

An *undulant fever* consists of periods of temperature elevation (usually lasting for days) alternated with afebrile periods (usually lasting for a week or more).

Children, the elderly and the very ill may not exhibit a febrile response to infection. In old people especially, an abrupt elevation of their normal temperature may be significant – even though 37 °C is not exceeded.

When assessing a patient with a persisting pyrexia, a full history is essential, with particular regard to possible relevant contacts, previous illnesses, immunizations, occupation, pets, current drug therapy and travel abroad. If the patient has been to areas in Africa where dangerous viral haemorrhagic fevers are present and there is no obvious diagnosis, specialist advice should be obtained after assessing the patient. The history should be followed by a complete examination, including a rectal and vaginal examination if there are no diagnostic symptoms or signs elsewhere. If there are no such clues, it is important to have established rapport with the patient, to explain the need for further tests, and to ask tactfully what he or she thinks is wrong – the replies are always interesting and sometimes informative!

Before commencing further investigations, there are two possible diagnoses to be considered.

(1) *Drug Fever.* Virtually any drug may cause fever without any other sign of drug intolerance. Temporary withdrawal of the suspected drug should be considered.

(2) *Factitious Fever.* This may be suspected from the demeanour of the patient, rapid defervescences in the absence of sweating, the lack of appropriate tachycardia, or (in those with a history of chronic fever) absence of weight loss. Continuously supervised temperature recordings, both rectal and oral, are necessary. Rapid post-voiding measurement of urinary temperature should reveal a temperature within 1.0–1.5 °C of the simultaneous oral temperature, or within 2 °C of the simultaneous rectal temperature: readings outside these limits are highly suggestive of factitious fever (Murray *et al.*, 1977. *N. Engl. J. Med.*, **296**, 23).

The encyclopaedic classification of disorders that may be responsible for persisting pyrexias is rather tedious, but some clarification is afforded by considering possible sites of pathology and the possible pathologies in turn.

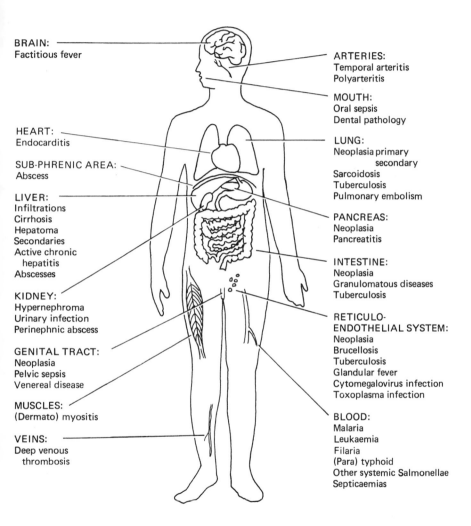

BRAIN:
Factitious fever

ARTERIES:
Temporal arteritis
Polyarteritis

MOUTH:
Oral sepsis
Dental pathology

HEART:
Endocarditis

LUNG:
Neoplasia primary
         secondary
Sarcoidosis
Tuberculosis
Pulmonary embolism

SUB-PHRENIC AREA:
Abscess

LIVER:
Infiltrations
Cirrhosis
Hepatoma
Secondaries
Active chronic
  hepatitis
Abscesses

PANCREAS:
Neoplasia
Pancreatitis

INTESTINE:
Neoplasia
Granulomatous diseases
Tuberculosis

KIDNEY:
Hypernephroma
Urinary infection
Perinephnic abscess

RETICULO-
ENDOTHELIAL SYSTEM:
Neoplasia
Brucellosis
Tuberculosis
Glandular fever
Cytomegalovirus infection
Toxoplasma infection

GENITAL TRACT:
Neoplasia
Pelvic sepsis
Venereal disease

MUSCLES:
(Dermato) myositis

VEINS:
Deep venous
  thrombosis

BLOOD:
Malaria
Leukaemia
Filaria
(Para) typhoid
Other systemic Salmonellae
Septicaemias

Figure 34   Sites where the aetiology of persistent pyrexias may remain hidden

The possible sites where 'classical pathology' may reside with few symptoms or signs are detailed in Figure 34.

141

Table 7   Infections which may present as a persistent pyrexia

Infection	Major illnesses	Useful clues or stigmata
SPECIFIC TO VARIOUS ORGANS	Diverticulitis Other bowel pathology	Past or present abnormal bowel habit
	Cholangitis	Hepatic tenderness, previous biliary colic or surgery
	Endocarditis	Change in heart murmur, emboli, microscopic haematuria
	Liver abscess	Hepatomegaly, rib tenderness, raised right diaphragm
	Mycoplasma pneumonia	Patchy CXR changes – more extensive than clinical signs suggest
	Osteomyelitis	Bone swelling, heat or tenderness
	Perinephric abscess	Septic focus elsewhere, IVP changes
	Psittacosis	Contact with (sick) birds
	Subphrenic abscess	Raised immobile right diaphragm
	Urinary tract infection	Abnormal ward urine test(s). Loin tenderness.
NOT SPECIFIC TO VARIOUS ORGANS	Brucellosis	Splenomegaly and/or lymphadenopathy. Contact with cattle or their products
	Cytomegalovirus infection	Atypical lymphocytes. Immunosuppressed patient
	Glandular fever	Sore throat, lymphadenopathy, splenomegaly, atypical lymphocytes
	Indigenous infections	History of travel from specific areas
	Leptospirosis	Occupational history, contact with rat infested areas, meningismus, jaundice with renal impairment
	Malaria	Sudden onset fever, rigors, headache. Splenomegaly
	Q fever	Contact with farm animals
	Secondary syphilis	Prior primary chancre. Copper coloured non-pruritic rash
	Septicaemias	Embolic lesions, purpura, focus for infection
	Toxoplasmosis	Lymphadenopathy
	Typhoid or paratyphoid fever	Rose spots, splenomegaly, dry cough, headache, constipation, usually travel abroad.

The major infectious syndromes which may present as fever of uncertain origin are detailed in Table 7.

Tuberculosis has a slowly progressive 'insidious' pathology and may cause persistent pyrexia with few focal symptoms or signs. The sites from which tuberculosis may cause a persistent pyrexia are listed in Table 8.

The major causes of persistent pyrexia not related to infection are detailed in Table 9.

Obviously these are daunting lists of possibilities and it would be impractical to proceed steadily through such lists excluding each diagnosis in turn. In the absence of leading symptoms or signs no matter how 'trivial',

Table 8   Sites from which tuberculosis may present as a persistent pyrexia

Situation	Useful clues or stigmata
Bone	X-ray of abnormal bones, positive Mantoux
Central nervous system	Gradual onset of cerebral dysfunction
Gut	Abdominal pain (especially in immigrants)
Joints	Aspiration and Ziehl–Nielsen stain
Lungs	Apical changes, cavitation/calcification, associated fluffy shadowing. Miliary mottling
Peritoneum	Abdominal pain, ascites, especially in immigrants
Urinary tract	Usually no early findings except sterile pyuria. May present as renal colic. Often seen in otherwise fit patients

Table 9   Major non-infectious causes of persistent pyrexia

	Site or illness	Useful clues or stigmata
NEOPLASMS WITH A TENDENCY TO BE OCCULT	Gut	Faecal occult bloods positive (?reliability of test) abdominal pain, change in bowel habit
	Hodgkin's disease + reticuloses in general	Negative Mantoux, itching, lymphadenopathy, Pel–Ebstein type undulant fever
	Leukaemias	Blood film usually diagnostic, if not marrow is
	Lung	CXR (PA and lateral) usually suggestive
	Renal	Haematuria in some cases, renal swelling on plain X-ray of abdomen or IVP
	Hepatic primary or secondaries	Arterial bruit, hepatic rub, raised alkaline phosphatase, irregular hepatomegaly
COLLAGEN DISEASES	Systemic lupus erythematosus	Butterfly rash, polyarthritis, leukopenia (especially if present in young females), LE cells and antinuclear factor positive
	Polyarteritis nodosa	Infarctive lesions, arterial thickenings, leukocytosis
	Rheumatic fever	Carditis, nodules, migratory polyarthritis
	Rheumatoid arthritis	Characteristic joint involvement
	Still's disease	Characteristic joint involvement, suggestive rash
INFLAMMATORY DISEASES ? AETIOLOGY	Crohn's disease	Right iliac fossa pain and/or swelling
	Sarcoidosis	Negative Mantoux, hilar lymphadenopathy on CXR
	Ulcerative colitis	Bloody/mucousy/pussy diarrhoea. Inflamed rectal mucosa on proctoscopy
OTHER DISORDERS	Aetiocholanolone fever	Diagnostic desperation!
	Drug fever	Administration of virtually any drug

143

Table 9 (cont).

Site or illness	Useful clues or stigmata
Factitious fever	No loss of weight with a prolonged fever, rapid defervescence without sweating, discrepancy between oral, rectal and urine temperatures
Pulmonary embolism	Calf pains, dyspnoea without obvious explanation, electrocardiogram changes. CXR changes if present
Familial Mediterranean fever	Recurrent abdominal pains. Ethnic origin, family history

'minor' or 'incidental', one should obviously perform sensible investigations restricted by the knowledge that, in an individual patient, there is no such thing as a differential diagnosis – there is usually only one correct diagnosis and a host of wrong diagnoses. The following would seem a sensible preliminary screen.

(1) *Haemoglobin*: most chronic febrile illnesses are associated with an anaemia, often normochromic and normocytic initially, with the subsequent possibility of hypochromia even in the absence of chronic blood loss: the serum iron and iron binding capacity are usually both low. The anaemia of chronic disorders rarely falls below 9 g/dl in the absence of blood loss or haemolysis.

(2) *White Cell Count*: this may be high in most extracellular infections causing fever. It may be low in intracellular infections (e.g. viruses, tuberculosis and brucellosis) and there may be a relative or absolute lymphocytosis.

(3) *Blood film examination with appropriate stains*: this may reveal pancytopenia secondary to leukaemia, malaria or bone marrow dysfunction. Toxic granulation of the white cells is often found in infections.

(4) *Cultures*:
   (a) of the blood even if the patient is afebrile as the very young, the very old or the very ill may be septicaemic yet apyrexial,
   (b) of the throat,
   (c) of the faeces,
   (d) of the urine (also look for the microscopic haematuria of infective endocarditis) and
   (e) of any other discharge.
   Consider asking specifically for Ziehl–Nielsen stain and cultures for tuberculosis.

(5) *Urea and electrolytes*: although of physiological help, they are rarely of diagnostic assistance.

144

(6) *Serum bilirubin*: this is raised in hepatocellular dysfunction, haemolysis and biliary stasis which may be caused by either hepatitis or mechanical biliary tract obstruction. If indicated, request measurement of both conjugated and unconjugated bilirubin.

(7) *Aspartate transaminase*: this is elevated in liver cell damage, muscle damage (both heart and skeletal) and lung damage. It may be slightly elevated if there is haemolysis.

(8) *Alkaline phosphatase*: this is raised in the presence of new bone formation, irritated biliary epithelium (even if jaundice is absent) and the placenta of pregnant women.

(9) *Erythrocyte sedimentation rate*: if very high, say in excess of 40–50 mm/h, think of generalized bacterial infections, mycoplasma infection with associated cold agglutinins, tuberculosis, collagen-vascular diseases, uraemia and malignancies – especially myeloma in the elderly.

(10) *Chest X-ray*: for evidence of intrathoracic disease not evident clinically.

(11) *Plain X-ray of the abdomen*: for evidence of hepatic or splenic enlargement, gallstones, pancreatic calcification, absent psoas shadows and other anatomical abnormalities.

(12) *A first specimen of serum*: not necessarily for viral studies alone – subsequent developments may be elucidated by retrospective testing of various serum parameters.

(13) *Mantoux testing*: in British patients a strongly positive or paradoxically a negative Mantoux test in ill patients (especially in those who have been known to be Mantoux positive) are suggestive of tuberculosis. In patients in whom the Mantoux test is negative at high concentration consider the possibility of reticulosis (including Hodgkin's disease) and sarcoidosis, in both there is a failure to react to certain 'allergic' stimuli (anergy).

(14) *Electrocardiogram*: may reveal evidence of carditis or pulmonary embolism.

All the above are non-invasive, quickly performed and cause minimal discomfort to the patient. If diagnostic clues do not emerge and fever persists hospital admission to a unit with isolation facilities should be requested. Non-invasive procedures including scans and ultrasound may then be utilized, but usually invasive investigations such as barium and other contrast-medium studies, endoscopy, or biopsy of appropriate tissues are necessary. If there are still no diagnostic clues despite repeated history and examination (possibly with complete reclerking of the patient by an uninvolved colleague), then after a period of observation consideration should be given to diagnostic laparotomy: this period of observation serves to exclude the possibility of spontaneous resolution or the appearance of diagnostic clinical signs.

Throughout the various deliberations, it is essential that the patient be kept fully informed so that his confidence in management is maintained despite the absence of a diagnosis. A non-factitious patient must not be allowed to suspect factitious doctoring!

Treatment

Particularly in immigrants, there may be a strong clinical suspicion of tuberculosis but the organism may not be visualized on Ziehl–Nielsen stain and, whilst awaiting the results of culture (which may take up to 6 weeks), a therapeutic trial of antituberculous therapy may be indicated – particularly with drugs such as isoniazid and ethambutol which have no activity against other bacteria. If a 'diagnostic' response occurs 'classical' triple therapy should be instituted.

If factitious fever is confirmed or suspected, the patient should receive appropriate psychiatric help. A diagnosis of factitious fever should not have to be a diagnosis of exclusion: on two occasions this author confirmed clinical suspicion by the use of the following question: 'I know a few of the temperature recordings are not genuine, but what I would *really* (Lies, all lies!) like to know is how frequent are the sweating attacks?' A numerical reply without rebuttal of the initial provisional clause implies factitious fever.

Overall in most 'classically defined' pyrexias of unknown origin, infections are diagnosed in about 40%, neoplasms in about 20% and collagen-vascular diseases in about 15% of cases.

FEBRILE PATIENTS FROM THE TROPICS AND SUBTROPICS

Tropical medicine textbooks contain details of numerous bizarre infections which are rarely, if at all, imported into Britain. Most imported infections are of common tropical diseases and, with the exception of certain dangerous African derived viral haemorrhagic fevers (VHF), diagnosis and treatment should be relatively easy once the common 'British' causes of persistent pyrexia seem unlikely. Figures 35–42 show the world distribution of some common tropical diseases.

In a patient who has recently returned from abroad it is essential that a full dated history of travel and activities is taken, including the diseases with which he is known to have been in contact, the general hygienic conditions to which he was exposed and details of the pre-visit immunizations and any prophylaxis taken whilst abroad.

The incubation periods of various tropical diseases related to the timing of travel obviously influence diagnostic possibilities (Table 10). In general, most infectious illnesses which have a rapidly progressive course after onset have an incubation period of less than 1 month.

Table 10 Diseases possibly acquired in the tropics; incubation periods

The disease	The time within which a patient cannot develop the illness after entering an at risk area (i.e. minimum incubation period)	The maximum period during which a patient can develop an illness after leaving an at risk area (i.e. maximum incubation period)	Average incubation period
PULMONARY EMBOLISM	0		
LASSA FEVER	3 days	17 days[1]	6–14 days
MARBURG VIRUS DISEASE	3 days	9 days[1]	
RELAPSING FEVER	3 days	about 18 days	7 days
YELLOW FEVER	3 days	15 days	3–6 days
EBOLA VIRUS DISEASE	4 days	17 days[1]	about 10 days
LEPTOSPIROSIS	4 days	19 days	about 12 days
MURINE TYPHUS	6 days	14 days	10–12 days
SCRUB TYPHUS	6 days	21 days	
BRUCELLOSIS	7 days	?	
TYPHOID	7 days	variable	8–14 days
TICK TYPHUS	7 days	18 days	about 12 days
SMALLPOX	7 days	17 days	10–12 days
FALCIPARUM MALARIA	8 days	25 days[2] (in non-immunes, longer in immunes)	12 days
VIVAX MALARIA	8 days	27 days[2] (in non-immunes, much longer in immunes)	14 days
EPIDEMIC TYPHUS	8 days	15 days	12 days
OVALE MALARIA	9 days	17 days[2] (in non-immunes)	15 days
Q FEVER	9 days	20 days	14 days
PRIMARY SYPHILIS	10 days	90 days	21 days
KALA AZAR	10 days	2 years	2–4 months
AMOEBIASIS	A few days–14 days	variable	
TRYPANOSOMIASIS (rhodesiense)	14 days	21 days	
MALARIAE MALARIA	15 days	30 days[2] (in non-immunes, much longer in immunes. Late relapses years later)	
HEPATITIS A	15 days	40 days	28 days

[1] = DHSS limits 3–21 days. [2] = prophylaxis may greatly extend

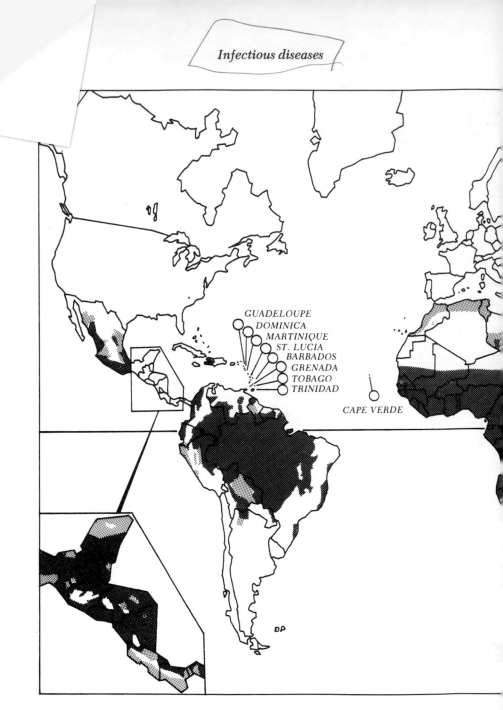

Figure 35 World distribution of malaria (1977). Data from WHO weekly Epidemiological Record, **52**, 344

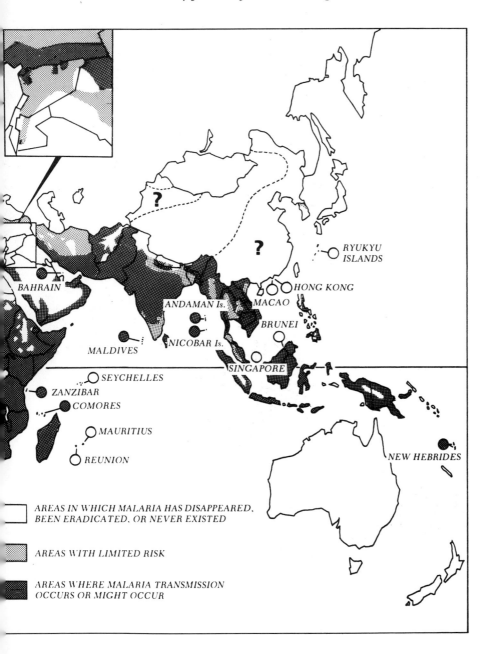

AREAS IN WHICH MALARIA HAS DISAPPEARED,
BEEN ERADICATED, OR NEVER EXISTED

AREAS WITH LIMITED RISK

AREAS WHERE MALARIA TRANSMISSION
OCCURS OR MIGHT OCCUR

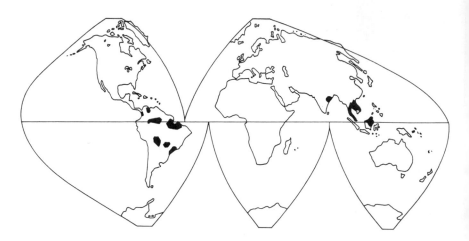

Figure 36   World distribution of chloroquine-resistant *P. falciparum* malaria

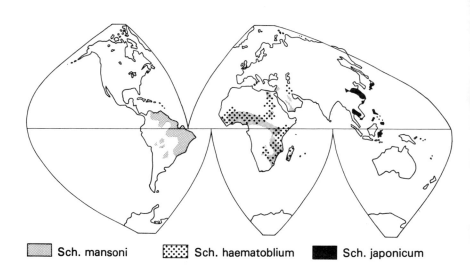

Sch. mansoni   Sch. haematoblium   Sch. japonicum

Figure 37   World distribution of schistosomiasis

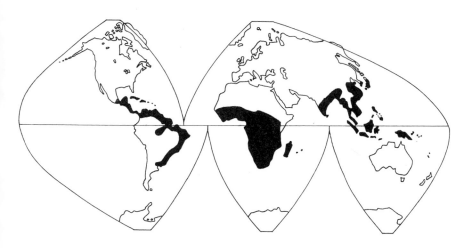

Figure 38 World distribution of filariasis

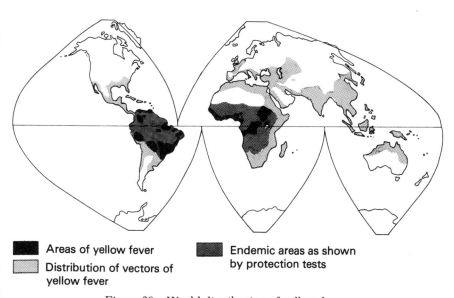

Areas of yellow fever

Distribution of vectors of yellow fever

Endemic areas as shown by protection tests

Figure 39 World distribution of yellow fever

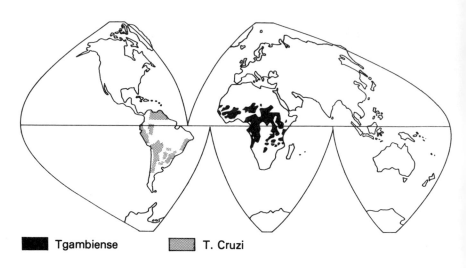

Figure 40   World distribution of trypanosomiasis

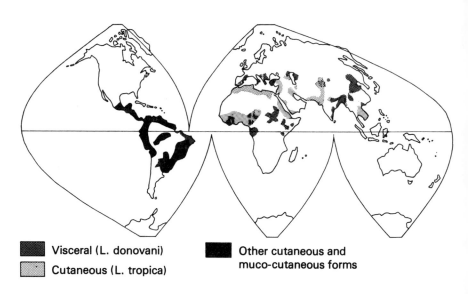

Figure 41   World distribution of leishmaniasis

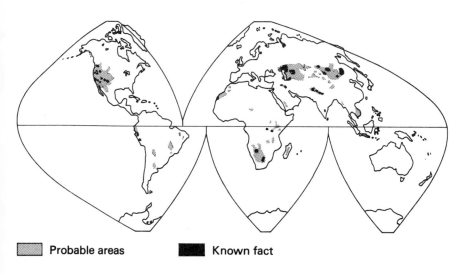

Probable areas   Known fact

Figure 42   World distribution of plague

Causes of fever which may occur within a month of travel in the Tropics or Subtropics

Falciparum malaria

This protozoan parasite is common in South-East Asia, Africa and tropical regions of the American continents: it is a killer disease which is both preventable and treatable. Although called malignant *tertian* malaria initially the fever commonly has no characteristic pattern, but it certainly may be malignant, being responsible for almost all of the malaria deaths that occur in Britain. Regular ingestion of malarial prophylaxis does *not* exclude the possibility of malaria but may extend the incubation period.

Falciparum malaria may present as an 'encephalitic' illness, a gastro-enteritic illness, a febrile jaundice or a shock syndrome. Given such a variety of presentations it is *essential* that any febrile patient from a malaria endemic area has malaria excluded. Diagnosis requires only an appropriately stained blood film and treatment of an early case is relatively simple: remember that in some parts of South-East Asia and South America there is chloroquine-resistant malaria and that quinine or Fansidar is required for treatment.

Other types of malaria may present with virtually any incubation period, particularly if ineffective prophylaxis has been taken.

153

Typhoid

Typhoid is usually an imported infection. Initially symptoms other than feverishness may be vague but abdominal discomfort, splenomegaly, constipation and dry cough are suggestive. Rose spots if seen are also suggestive. Cultures of blood, urine and stool should be performed. The history of recent immunization and the Widal test result may be interesting but should not influence one's diagnostic thoughts. As soon as the diagnosis is confirmed or even before if the diagnosis is likely, this disease should be notified by telephone to the relevant community physician.

Non-typhoidal Salmonella infections

These may present as febrile illnesses, especially if there is bloodstream invasion. Usually, but not always, there are gastrointestinal symptoms.

Hepatitis

Both hepatitis A and B may present in the prodromal period as a febrile illness with constitutional upset and the urine may contain excess urobilinogen or bilirubin. Yellow fever is a possibility in non-vaccinated patients who have visited tropical Africa or tropical regions of the American continent within the previous 3–15 days.

Leptospirosis

If severe may produce Weil's syndrome with a sudden onset of fever, headache, meningism, a rash, haemorrhagic lesions, jaundice or conjunctival injection. A raised white cell count, urea or ESR are all suggestive. However, the spectrum of illness is quite wide and diagnosis may have to rely on blood and urine studies and serological tests.

Typhus

Suspicion usually occurs if there is an eschar or if the patient is known to have visited endemic or epidemic areas. With the exception of louse borne classical typhus these infections are not transmissible in Britain; the vectors are not indigenous to Britain and are not usually carried by the patient.

Relapsing fever

Louse borne relapsing fever is usually acquired in Africa, whereas tick borne relapsing fever has a wider geographical distribution including areas in the Near East, Southern USSR, the Mediterranean basin, Africa, Southern USA and South America. The illness has spontaneous remissions and relapses.

Viral infections

There are many viral infections which may give rise to mild febrile illnesses. Care should be exercised in dealing with such patients' blood and bodily fluids as a patient in this category may occasionally have a dangerous transmissible infection. The management of feverish patients from Africa, who fall into a separate category, is detailed later.

Venereal disease

Secondary syphilis and gonococcal septicaemia are possible diseases of travellers, who may have continued to experience 'home comforts' whilst abroad.

Pulmonary embolism

Deserves special mention as travel by aeroplane implies prolonged pressure on and stasis within the leg venous system, which can lead to thrombosis with subsequent pulmonary emboli.

Causes of tropical fever which may occur at any time after return to Britain

Malaria

Especially *P. vivax, ovale* and *malariae,* but also *P. falciparum* (particularly if ineffective prophylaxis had been taken).

Hepatitis B

Both acute hepatitis and the HBs Ag carrier state are common in the tropics. Symptoms and signs are similar to hepatitis A but the onset of hepatitis B is said to be more insidious and prodromal rashes and arthralgia are also more common in hepatitis B.

Tuberculosis

Immigrants in particular may present with occult tuberculosis as a cause for fever. In some instances, the focus may be found but in others no focus may be identified and the diagnosis has to be made and confirmed by response to antituberculous therapy. Miliary tuberculosis may have few if any physical signs and a *negative* Mantoux test is suggestive (as if sensitivity to tuberculoprotein is 'mopped up' by the infection, or perhaps an 'idiopathic' insensitivity allowed tuberculosis to become rampant). The diagnosis is almost certain if the Mantoux test becomes positive after a period of antituberculous therapy.

Amoebiasis

Invasive amoebiasis, including metastatic spread, may present at any time in patients who have visited the tropics.

With metastatic amoebiasis, history or evidence of amoebic colitis may not be present at presentation. Amoebic liver abscesses usually present with fever, an enlarged, tender liver with pain on percussion of overlying ribs. Both the white cell count and ESR are usually elevated: the right diaphragm may be raised and relatively immobile clinically and on X-ray. Serological tests, including the fluorescent antibody test, are positive in about 95% of cases.

Amoebic colitis may be mistaken for ulcerative colitis with disastrous results if steroids are utilized.

Invasive worm infections

If presenting with a brief febrile illness these infections usually have an associated eosinophilia.

Imported trypanosomiasis

The parasite is almost always African in derivation. A chancre may be present, or have been noted by the patient: progressive decline in cerebral function, hepatosplenomegaly and lymph node enlargement may be evident. Diagnosis is by identification of the organism in appropriately stained blood films, lymph node aspirates or by serological tests.

Visceral leishmaniaisis (Kala-azar)

If well developed there will be fever, liver enlargement, splenic enlargement and pancytopenia.

FEBRILE PATIENTS WHO HAVE LEFT AFRICA WITHIN THE PREVIOUS THREE WEEKS

In addition to diseases previously mentioned there are three African viral haemorrhagic fevers (VHF) which require high security facilities for their investigation and containment – Lassa fever (LF), Ebola virus disease

(EVD) and Marburg virus disease (MVD).

Although a VHF suspect may be a risk to others, the main risk to the suspect is that a treatable illness (such as malaria) will not be diagnosed and treated expeditiously.

Plainly it is impossible to treat all patients from Africa as VHF suspects and the following details may be of help in differential diagnosis of such patients.

Lassa fever

It is likely that LF is present in most bush areas of West Africa. In parts of Liberia and Sierra Leone LF is endemic and there is serological evidence of LF in Nigeria, Ivory Coast, Mali, Central African Republic, Guinea and Eastern Senegal. LF is initially transmitted to humans via the urine of a bush rat (*Mastomyces natalensis*): this rat is not found in large cities and thus LF in general only affects patients who have been into bush areas. Despite hysteria to the contrary it appears that in the early stages patients are not highly infectious to the general public unless the sufferer has respiratory symptoms or signs. However, infection may easily be acquired from blood, urine and other bodily fluids and thus hospital workers and paramedical personnel may be at risk of nosocomial (hospital acquired) infection.

In recognized cases the incubation period has been 3–17 days. An insidious onset illness follows with a fever which usually persists for 7–17 days with chills, headache, myalgia, backache and malaise. A sore throat, with yellowish to white exudates and shallow ulcers on the pharynx, is characteristic. Prostration is classically out of proportion to the clinical signs including fever.

In the first week, vomiting and diarrhoea may occur. In the second week, tinnitus or deafness may occur and in a few patients a rash occurs 7–9 days after the onset of fever. Jaundice is *uncommon*, especially in the early stages. In severe infections, there is a rapid deterioration during the second week with signs of multiple organ dysfunction (all of the three VHFs are pantropic and thus damage most bodily tissues). The mortality of hospitalized cases up to 1975 was 45% but the community-based mortality is almost certainly much lower.

Ebola and Marburg virus disease

In 1967 Marburg virus disease caused a high mortality outbreak (approximately 24%) related to vervet monkeys exported from Uganda. In 1975 two people were infected by a patient who had acquired this infection from an unknown source in Rhodesia. The incubation period is 3–9 days.

A clinically similar but antigenically distinct illness, Ebola virus disease

(EVD), occurred in Northern Zaire and Southern Sudan in 1976, in which the mortality rate was about 65%. There was a similar high mortality epidemic in the same area in 1979. Airborne infection seemed unlikely, and the major spread was possibly due to infected blood or an insect vector. The incubation period was 4–17 days.

In both MVD and EVD there is a sudden onset of headache, retro-orbital pain, backache, prostration and fever which lasts about one week. Conjunctival injection is common. There may be generalized lymph node enlargement and hepatomegaly, although early jaundice is unusual. A few days after the onset, vomiting, abdominal pain and diarrhoea commence as may respiratory symptoms. Between days 4–7 a perifollicular, erythematous, non-irritating maculo-papular rash appears and other haemorrhagic phenomena may become apparent.

Early differentiation between these transmissible high mortality illnesses and other diseases is therefore necessary.

Who is at risk?

Lassa fever appears to be a disease of a fairly predictable geographical occurrence in West Africa. EVD and MVD almost certainly have animal reservoirs or vectors outside major cities and until these are identified it seems that one cannot regard any rural bush area in Africa as being entirely risk free. Hopefully small epidemics will be rapidly notified so that patients from these areas can be treated as suspects. However the occurrence of the 'sporadic' case of MVD in Rhodesia is worrying.

In Britain LF suspects are numerically the most common (Emond *et al.*, 1978; Galbraith *et al.*, 1978) and the following features may serve to diagnose more 'mundane' illnesses at an early stage, but one cannot of course exclude the possibility of coincidental VHF infection.

Diphtheria

This may cause oropharyngeal manifestations in a toxic ill patient.

Falciparum malaria

This illness, unlike LF, has an abrupt onset usually with early rigors, and if splenomegaly is present malaria is highly likely. Lymph node enlargement and skin rashes are most unusual in malaria.

Typhoid

It may be difficult to distinguish typhoid from LF as both may have insidious onset of fever, headache, backache, and respiratory or gastrointestinal symptoms. Sore throat is uncommon in early typhoid and its presence favours LF.

Typhus

Typhus usually has an abrupt onset of illness. Sore throat or gastrointestinal symptoms are not common.

Severe leptospirosis

There is usually a sudden onset with fever, severe myalgia, vomiting, albuminuria and evidence of bleeding: this is compatible with EVD or MVD. However, jaundice is rare in the early stages of VHF.

Yellow fever

The disease is unlikely if patients have been vaccinated but, as in EVD and MVD, illness may be of an abrupt onset. Despite the name, jaundice need not be a feature of illness. Bleeding may occur in yellow fever but there is no rash.

Influenza

Influenza has a fairly abrupt onset of symptoms.

It is not uncommon for recent arrivals in Britain to develop trivial transient feverish illnesses (presumably viral in aetiology), and this added to the fact that in Britain patients often present early in any illness means that details of the *late* symptoms and signs of various febrile illnesses are substantially unhelpful; hence preliminary management must be based on epidemiological evidence. The following criteria of risk assessment are suggested:

Minimal risk – Febrile patients who have stayed exclusively in major cities (in which the risks of VHF are negligible) within 3 weeks prior to illness can be treated as routine infectious disease patients.

Moderate risk – Patients who have visited small towns or country districts within 3 weeks prior to illness should be treated with more suspicion, and specialist advice sought from a consultant in Infectious Diseases.

High risk – Patients who have been living or working in rural areas, medical and nursing staff from country hospitals, contacts of known cases, and laboratory workers handling dangerous material within 3 weeks prior to the onset of illness should be treated with maximum suspicion, and investigated under high security facilities.

When presented with any patient in the latter two categories, reference should also be made to the 1976 Memorandum on Lassa Fever. If there is *any doubt* concerning management or investigation of a particular patient, *the investigation of choice is a telephone call* to a designated high security unit or a tropical disease centre seeking further advice.

REFERENCES

Emond, R.T.D., Smith, H. and Welsby P.D. (1978). *Br. Med. J.*, 1, 966

Galbraith, N.S., Berrie, J.R.H., Forbes, P. and Young, S. (1978). *J. R. Soc. Hlth.*, 98, 152

Suggested further reading

Daggett, P. (1976). A system for the investigation of pyrexia of unknown origin. *Br. J. Hosp. Med.*, 357

Murray, H.W., Tuazon, C.U., Guerrero, I.C., Claudio, M.S., Alling, D.W. and Sheagren, J.N. (1977). Urinary temperature: a clue to the early diagnosis of factitious fever. *N. Engl. J. Med.*, 296, 23

Petersdorf, R.G. and Bennett, I.L. (1957). Factitious fever. *Ann. Intern. Med.*, 46, 1039

11
Superficial manifestations of infectious diseases

Skin lesions are often the most noticeable accompaniment to infectious diseases, and diagnosis of the common three childhood infectious diseases which are associated with a rash — measles, rubella (German measles) and chickenpox — is relatively easy. Points of particular value in differential diagnosis are in italics.

Measles

This is a highly infectious disease which was, prior to vaccination, a 'routine' childhood illness. There is no carrier state. Infection is by droplet, direct contact, or airborne spread, and the incubation period is 8–11 days to the onset of fever, and about 12–14 days until the rash appears.

There is a *3–4 day prodrome* of fever, irritability and conjunctivitis: *respiratory tract misery* is prominent comprising rhinitis, coryza, laryngitis, tracheitis and bronchitis, often with a characteristic cough. Occasionally gastrointestinal symptoms may be prominent. The prodromal symptoms usually start to improve once the rash has erupted.

Koplik's spots are present during the prodrome: they are well-nigh pathognomonic of measles and may be found wherever there are mucous secreting glands, classically they occur adjacent to the molar teeth and

161

appear as 'coarse grains of salt on a background of red velvet'.

As the Koplik's spots are fading *the rash appears behind the ears*, on the face, and then *spreads from above downwards* to the body and limbs. The rash consists of dusky red macules or papules which may coalesce to form *irregular blotches*: these blanch on pressure. After 2–3 days the *rash fades in the same order as it evolved*, leaving transient brownish *staining* which lasts for less than a week. Staining does not blanch on pressure. Occasionally desquamation occurs. Infectivity is from the onset of the prodrome until staining has occurred.

Complications

These include secondary infection, particularly of the lungs and ears, and encephalitis. A thrombocytopenia may result, as may a haemorrhagic 'black' measles which possibly results from a severe vasculitis.

Treatment

Treatment is symptomatic with antibacterial therapy being reserved for bacterial infections: prophylactic antibacterial drugs are not indicated. Appropriate isolation is indicated. Remember that *any* patient given *any* drug during the measles prodrome will develop a measles, not drug induced, rash.

Rubella (German measles)

German measles is very infectious, but not all of those infected develop a rash. Previous rubella (and to a lesser extent vaccination) confers strong immunity to clinical illness but minor or subclinical illness may occur. The incubation period is 17–18 days, with a range of 14–21 days. The infective period is from 7 days before until 5 days after the rash appears. Infants with congenital rubella excrete the virus heavily for long periods of time. The clinical diagnosis of rubella is notoriously unreliable as various echo, coxsackie and adenoviruses can cause an indistinguishable illness. Measles or drug rashes may also be difficult to distinguish from rubella. For all practical purposes, a history of rubella unconfirmed by serology should be ignored.

A rash occurs more frequently in older children and adults. The rash consists of discrete delicate pink macules (very occasionally papular and haemorrhagic elements may be present) which may not evolve further or which may coalesce to form a pinkish flush resembling scarlet fever but *without puncta*. The rash *starts on the face and behind the ears*, and then *spreads from above downwards: staining is very unusual* and desquamation only occurs in severe cases.

There is *slight enlargement of lymph nodes, particularly of the suboccipital and posterior auricular groups*. There is no *coryza*, usually *no cough*, and *no Koplik's spots*. The eyes often feel gritty. The throat may be reddened but tonsillar exudates are uncommon.

Patients with measles are sicker, and their illness lasts for a longer time (another name for rubella is 3-day measles). Patients who have scarlet fever are generally more ill and have a raised white cell count.

Complications

Complications include *arthralgia/arthritis* (especially in young women) affecting the small joints of the hands and feet, encephalitis of variable severity, purpura or thrombocytopenia. Congenital rubella may occur in the infants of infected mothers (see Chapter 3).

Treatment

Treatment is symptomatic with appropriate isolation. There is no specific therapy for encephalitis.

Chickenpox (varicella)

In adults there may be a brief prodrome, but children often have the rash as the first manifestation of illness.

The rash consists of *one to five crops of vesicles* usually occurring over 1 week or less. Individual lesions start as macules or papules which progress (so rapidly that they are often unnoticed) to form *vesicles* that are markedly *pruritic*, superficial, unilocular and tend to be oval or elliptical. These develop into *pustules* which then crust. There is no scarring as long as the lesions are not scratched.

The distribution is *centripetal* (centre-seeking): flexor surfaces are favoured and axillary lesions may occur.

The enanthem consists of small intra-oral vesicles which usually break down to form shallow ulcers.

The incubation period is usually 14–18 days and the infective period is a few days before the rash appears until the last lesion has crusted – usually about 7 days after the last vesicle develops. Constitutional symptoms abate as the cropping ceases.

Complications

Complications include secondary bacterial infection of the skin or lungs, pneumonia due to varicella-zoster virus itself, and encephalitis: mild cerebellar disturbances are not uncommon. (I have observed that patients with chickenpox cannot stand on one leg with their eyes shut!)

Treatment

Treatment is symptomatic with appropriate isolation. Adenine arabinoside may have to be used for severe chickenpox in the immunocompromised.

The differential diagnosis includes impetigo (no enanthem), insect bites (which often possess urticarial elements unassociated with constitutional symptoms or enanthem) and scabies (in which burrows will be evident).

Differentiation from smallpox

Although the world has been declared free from smallpox, it is not impossible that the virus may escape from laboratories, be a mutation from genetically similar African viruses, or perhaps even be used as a germ warfare exercise. In contrast to chickenpox, the lesions of smallpox all erupted simultaneouly, were *deep set*, tended to be *circular* and were *multilocular*. There was a *longer, more severe prodrome*. The rash of smallpox was *centrifugal* (centre-fleeing), preferred extensor surfaces, and the axillae were often spared. Oral lesions occur in both smallpox and chickenpox.

If 'chickenpox' persists suspect dermatitis herpetiformis or pityriasis lichenoides varioliformis and obtain dermatological advice.

CUTANEOUS MANIFESTATIONS OF OTHER INFECTIOUS DISEASES

Shingles (Herpes-zoster)

This is caused by the varicella-zoster virus (which also causes chickenpox). Shingles is usually limited to one or more contiguous dermatomes and is almost invariably unilateral with a midline cut-off. Occasionally motor dysfunction can be an additional feature. If the rash appears to extend across the midlines the diagnosis of shingles is suspect, or secondary bacterial infection such as cellulitis has occurred.

The shingles eruption is somewhat like a simultaneous, dense, single crop of chicken pocks, in which groups of confluent vesicles occur, with an erythematous base and a distinct dermatome distribution. In most patients with shingles, occasional chicken pocks may be seen with affected dermatome(s), but if the chicken pocks are extensive an underlying malignancy or immune defect becomes more suspect.

As a group, patients with shingles have rashes predominantly in a distribution pattern similar to individual cases of chickenpox – with thoracic, abdominal and cranial dermatomes being particularly affected. Given the pathogenesis (p. 58, Chapter 3) this may be a pathologically relevant comment.

Shingles is infectious in that chickenpox may develop in susceptibles.

164

Controversially it seems that shingles may occur after an initiating exposure to exogenous varicella-zoster virus.

Usually there is only slight constitutional disturbance, but in about 5% of patients there is fever, malaise, neck stiffness or nausea. Many patients experience prodromal pain or paraesthesiae in the dermatome(s) of the future eruption.

Complications

Complications include secondary bacterial infection, viral meningoencephalitis, and motor nerve dysfunction. Post-herpetic neuralgia may be severe and persistent. *Ophthalmic shingles*: Often patients experience prodromal pain on combing the hair. If the nasociliary nerve innervated area is affected serious eye complications are likely, including iridocyclitis, keratoconjunctivitis and chemosis. Treatment consists of mydriatic eye drops (in the absence of glaucoma) to dilate the pupil and thus prevent adhesions between the iris and the lens. Steroid and anti-bacterial eyedrops may have to be used. An ophthalmological opinion is advisable. *Geniculate shingles* (the Ramsay Hunt syndrome) presents with pain in the ear and throat with vesicles in the external auditory meatus. Often there is loss of sensation in the ipsilateral two thirds of the tongue, and paralysis of the facial nerve of the lower motor neurone type.

Treatment of shingles

Generally treatment is symptomatic, with appropriate isolation. Post-herpetic neuralgia may be a considerable problem, especially in the elderly. Non-narcotic analgesia should be used with assistance from tranquillizers or anti-depressants if required. Sometimes the antiepileptic drug carbamazepine is useful. Rarely, surgical procedures may be required. Topical 5-idoxuridine (in dimethyl sulphoxide as a penetrating agent) is of proven efficacy. I suspect that most patients in domiciliary practice will not continue the treatment because of the stinging of the topical preparation and the nauseating taste caused by the rapid absorption of the dimethyl sulphoxide.

Herpes simplex

There are two viruses which cause human infection:

Type 1 infections usually cause a trivial illness consisting of clusters of vesicles which usually last less than 10 days. Classically, lesions occur in or around the mouth (Herpes labialis or febrilis, 'cold sores') but lesions may occur elsewhere on the body. The vesicles often itch or cause a burning sensation. They may break down to leave superficial erosions – which heal without scarring. The eruption may be triggered by almost any stress, including other infections. Recurrent attacks are frequent. Various topical treatments are effective, including 5-idoxuridine, but mild attacks hardly require treatment.

Type 2 infections, in contrast to Type 1 infections, usually cause 'below the waist' eruptions, including vulvo-vaginitis and cervicitis (the latter being a predisposing factor to the subsequent development of carcinoma of the cervix). Severe Herpes simplex infections of both types may be treated with intravenous adenine arabinoside.

Other superficial manifestations of Herpes simplex infection include:

(1) *Acute generalized Herpes simplex*: a high mortality disease in neonates, who acquire infection (often Type 2) perinatally from the mother's birth canal. It is usually diagnosed at autopsy.

(2) *Erythema multiforme* or the more extensive Stevens–Johnson syndrome may follow *Herpes simplex* infection.

(3) *Herpetic eye infection* may have various manifestations including vesicles on the eyelids, coarse punctate epithelial opacities, iridocyclitis and superficial dendritic corneal ulcers (best seen after fluorescein staining). Steroid therapy is contraindicated.

(4) *Skin infection* may be extensive, particularly in those with eczema. Recovery is often surprisingly good, possibly because eczema herpeticum lesions are smaller and more superficial than those of eczema vaccinatum (caused by vaccinia virus). The term Kaposi's varicelliform eruption is used to describe extensive eczema herpeticum or eczema vaccinatum.

(5) *Herpetic whitlows* are caused by implantation of Herpes simplex virus. They tend to be an occupation-related diseases of dentists, doctors, nurses and others involved with oral care. There is no pus formation and incision is valueless. Topical 5-idoxuridine speeds recovery.

Echo viruses, Coxsackie viruses and adenoviruses

Each may cause rashes with maculopapular or petechial elements: the rashes may resemble measles, rubella or scarlet fever. Occasionally vesicular or bullous lesions may result. The features of the associated illness may give diagnostically suggestive clues to these viral infections but often clinical diagnosis is difficult if not impossible.

Erythema infectiosum (fifth disease)

This begins as a marked erythema of the cheeks (the 'slapped cheek' appearance). 1–4 days later maculopapular lesions occur on the extremities and trunk. These assume a characteristic reticular pattern as they fade. The cause is unknown but is presumed to be a virus.

Hand, foot and mouth disease

This is usually caused by infection with a Coxsackie A virus. There is a mild illness, perhaps with a low grade fever, in which small vesicles occur on the hands, the feet, and in the mouth: in the mouth the appearances are those of herpangina – the vesicles break down to form small erosions or ulcers. There may be small epidemics among close contacts.

Infectious mononucleosis

This may give rise to a pinkish maculopapular eruption of patchy distribution with a predilection for extensor surfaces. Other stigmata of infectious mononucleosis may be present, including the typical throat appearances, lymph node enlargement or splenomegaly. The majority of patients given ampicillin or its derivatives will develop a rash – an undesirable but useful diagnostic occurrence. A pitfall in diagnosing infectious mononucleosis is the finding of biological false positive standard tests for syphilis: however the more specific treponemal antibody tests will be negative.

The two other agents that may cause a 'heterophil antibody negative' infectious mononucleosis syndrome may also cause rashes. Cytomegalovirus rashes occur most often in neonates with congenitally acquired disease: petechial, purpuric, diffuse papular or vesiculopapular rashes may occur. Toxoplasmosis may cause purpuric or maculopapular rashes.

Mucocutaneous lymph node syndrome (Kawasaki syndrome)

This is a presumed (viral) infection common in Japan but currently uncommon in the United Kingdom. Patients are usually less than 2 years old. There is 1–2 weeks of fever with conjunctival injection, with dryness and redness of the lips, tongue and oropharynx. A red maculopapular rash occurs on day 3–5 of illness. There is tender non-suppurating lymph node enlargement, and often non-pitting oedema of the palms and soles. Subsequent skin peeling around the nail folds is highly suggestive of this syndrome. The prognosis is usually good but about 2% of children develop an illness resembling infantile polyarteritis with attendant morbidity and mortality.

Roseola infanticum (exanthem subitum or sixth disease)

This is a disease of infants and young children. There is 3–5 days of high fever and then a rubella-like rash when the fever falls. The face and lower limbs are usually spared and there is no staining. There are no Koplik's spots.

Smallpox

As the world will soon be *officially* smallpox-free, smallpox is likely to be forgotten. However, workers in smallpox laboratories or their contacts may contract smallpox. Such laboratory workers will presumably be vaccinated and less like to become ill, although they could still transmit the disease.

Vaccinia (smallpox vaccination)

Because smallpox vaccination will soon be limited to certain at-risk groups, infections with vaccinia and its complications will only occur in these groups *and* (by accidental transmission) amongst their close contacts. Complications of vaccination include allergic rashes, ectopic self-inoculation and post-vaccination encephalitis related either to a toxic encephalopathy or to perivenous demyelination. Three other complications are:

Eczema vaccinatum. Vaccinia spreads over large areas of eczematous skin. Patients may be infected by (negligent) vaccination or by close contact with a recently vaccinated person.

Generalized vaccinia consists of widespread lesions over the whole body, implying blood borne dissemination of vaccinia virus. It may be a severe illness, particularly in those with impaired immune responses.

Progressive vaccinia occurs when the patient's immune system fails to control the infection: the lesions continue to enlarge and spread whilst fresh lesions occur. Antibody deficiency (hypogammaglobulinaemia) may be one treatable cause.

Erysipelas

There is an acute onset of fever and spreading erythematous swelling of the skin: there is local heat and the infected area has a sharply defined border. Erysipelas, unlike shingles, does not respect dermatomes. The causative organism is almost invariably a penicillin sensitive streptococcus.

Impetigo

Impetigo is usually a childhood infection. Streptococcal impetigo causes gold yellow crusts, whereas staphylococcal impetigo often has superficial blisters which then burst and crust. Impetigo may complicate other skin diseases.

In an individual child, lesions may spread rapidly to all parts of the body: scratching fingers play a major role in transmission and child-to-child spread may be rapid.

Despite theoretical objections, topical antibacterial agents are effective in *trivial well circumscribed* impetigo. Widespread infection demands systemic antibacterial therapy, preferably administered parenterally. Children should be kept off school and should not play with friends until the infection has resolved.

With certain strains of staphylococci (especially phage type 71) toxic epidermal necrolysis may result, a condition in which the skin peels off to resemble scaled skin; the causative staphylococcus is usually penicillinase producing and thus penicillin is ineffective. Nikolski's sign is positive, i.e. by exerting lateral traction, with a finger, the skin slides at the periphery of a lesion.

In neonates extensive bullous impetigo may occur, the so-called pemphigus neonatorum.

Henoch-Schönlein purpura

This has a peak incidence between 2 and 5 years of age. It is vasculitis, commonly an allergic reaction to streptococcal infection. Classically the rash is a maculopapular purpuric eruption on the buttocks and extensor surfaces of the limbs. The rash appearances may range from a few petechiae-like lesions (which may be confused with those of meningococcal septicaema) to small haemorrhagic blisters. There may be associated arthritis (often of large joints and often migratory), abdominal pain with or without gastrointestinal bleeding, intussusception of involved areas of the bowel, and renal involvement. Treatment depends on the cause.

Leptospirosis

Occasionally, petechial and macular skin rashes occur. Suspect this diagnosis in those occupationally exposed to animals, especially if there is jaundice, a raised blood urea, and myalgia in association with a raised white cell count or raised erythrocyte sedimentation rate.

Scarlet fever

Scarlet fever is at present relatively uncommon in the United Kingdom. It is usually caused by infection with an erythrogenic toxin-producing strain of Lancefield Group A β-haemolytic streptococcus. Only certain strains can cause scarlet fever, but as these strains are transmissible scarlet fever is infectious. Immunity to the toxin is gained after an attack, and thus further attacks are unusual. Classically the throat is the site of the initiating infection, but occasionally infection of the skin or the cervix may be responsible. The incubation period is 2–4 days with a range of 1–7 days. The infective period is about 10–21 days after the onset, but this is shortened by antibacterial therapy.

Clinically there is an abrupt onset of fever, sore throat, and perhaps vomiting, in association with a streptococcal sore throat. The rash follows 24–36 hours later: there is a deep facial flush with relative circumoral pallor: the rash appears on the neck and spreads downwards as a 'lobster-red' erythema with tiny red points superimposed (punctate erythema).

The tongue is aptly described to have a white then red 'strawberry' appearance. The florid rash lasts 2–3 days and then starts to fade. Towards the end of the first week of illness the skin may peel in the same sequence as the rash evolved, therefore terminating at the hands and feet. This desquamation is very suggestive, but not pathognomonic, of scarlet fever.

Syphilis

Secondary syphilis may cause a non-irritant, copper coloured rash in which there may be both macular and papular elements: there may be associated constitutional symptoms. In *any* atypical 'infectious disease' rash syphilitic serology should be performed. Homosexuals are at particular risk of syphilis. In tertiary syphilis gummas may present as nodular or squamous lesions which are destructive, painless, indurated and chronic. If ulceration occurs a clean looking punched out ulcer results.

Cutaneous tuberculosis (Lupus vulgaris)

This is a brownish red papule or plaque which may ulcerate or scar over. Cutaneous tuberculosis may be suspected if ulcers develop in atypical places and then fail to heal spontaneously.

Skin rashes associated with septicaemias

Any febrile patient with an unexplained rash should have blood cultures performed. Most septicaemias can give rise to cutaneous manifestations.

Meningococcal septicaemia

This may give rise to characteristic petechiae or large ecchymotic areas, or both.

Staphylococcal septicaemia

Staphylococcal septicaemia is invariably a serious condition, and secondary localization may cause problems such as perinephric abscesses or osteomyelitis. Normal heart valves may be attacked and endocarditis produced.

Endocarditis

Cutaneous manifestations (which may not have time to develop before death in an acute endocarditis) include clubbing, splinter haemorrhages, Osler's nodes and Janeway lesions, generalized pigmentation and purpura.

Gonococcaemia

Typically there are a few haemorrhagic pustules, frequently found on the extremities, particularly on the fingers.

Listeria monocytogenes septicaemia

Red macules may be seen which undergo central necrosis with pustule formation.

Typhoid and paratyphoid fever

These infections (especially Paratyphi B) may cause crops of non-pruritic macules which blanch on pressure, and which normally occur on the trunk or chest. They are initiated by microemboli of the organism. Unless searched for specifically they are easy to miss, especially in the dark skinned. Similar lesions may occur in ornithosis.

Erythema multiforme

This consists of multiformed erythematous lesions, some of which have concentric haloes – the so-called target lesions. Some lesions may have a bullous centre. Erythema multiforme can be considered to be a reaction pattern with a variety of underlying causes, including Herpes simplex infection, mycoplasma infection, and drug allergy – particularly to penicillins, sulphonamides or barbiturates. Treatment is that of the cause if possible, or withdrawal of relevant drugs.

In the severe form of erythema multiforme, the Stevens–Johnson syndrome, there are additional mucosal lesions of the mouth, eyes and genitalia.

The manifestations usually last about 2 weeks. Steroids may hasten improvement but may have uncertain effects on underlying infections.

Erythema nodosum

This consists of spontaneously occurring painful reddish nodular 'bruise-like' lesions which commonly occur on the shins. The three common causes in the United Kingdom are streptococcal infections (do throat swab and

171

antistreptolysin O titre), sarcoidosis (hilar lymph node enlargement on chest X-ray?), and tuberculosis (Mantoux test suggestively positive? – if the Mantoux test is negative this is a pointer towards sarcoidosis).

Other causes include drug allergies, granulomatous diseases (leprosy, ulcerative colitis and Crohn's disease), syphilis, some fungal infections, certain viral infections, and underlying malignancy. Ulcerative colitis or Crohn's disease may cause a somewhat related eruption – pyoderma gangrenosum – in which there are irregular patches resembling primary infective foci, but with considerable necrosis at the centre. The lesions may commence as groups of pustules or as erythema nodosum-like lesions.

Erythema marginatum

This is almost pathognomonic of rheumatic fever. There is a rapidly-spreading, ringed eruption, occasionally with raised margins, which coalesce into annular patterns. The individual lesions resemble defibrillator burns.

Focal skin sepsis

Boils, carbuncles and other focal infective lesions are often caused by invasive strains of staphylococci or by impaired host defence mechanisms. Septicaemia may ensue. Metastatic skin lesions may occur by finger transfer after scratching.

Initial treatment should be with antibacterial agents that are not inactivated by penicillinase. These patients are an infection risk on general wards and should be discharged if possible, or nursed in appropriate isolation.

Superficial fungal infections

Superficial fungal infections are dealt with in Chapter 4.

CUTANEOUS MANIFESTATIONS OF OTHER AETIOLOGIES

Parasites

Fleas

Papular urticaria is a common sign of flea infestation: an afebrile patient has the continual appearance of pleomorphic, intensely itchy wheals which are surrounded by inflammation.

Lice

Infestation with *pediculus humanus corporis*, *capitis*, or *Phthirus pubis* (body lice, head lice, or crab lice respectively). Often the diagnosis is made by seeing the eggs or the lice themselves: one can look for minutes before focusing on a louse, but after *one* louse has been seen a horrifying number immediately becomes visible. Lice may cause small red papular lesions, perhaps with tiny central blood clots and occasionally with urticaria, thickening or discolouration of the skin.

Scabies

Human scabies causes intense irritation and maculopapular skin lesions. Interestingly, skin irritation only occurs after sensitization has taken place (usually one or more months after primary infection). Ninety per cent of patients have burrows visible in the interdigital spaces, and on the flexor surfaces of the wrists or elbows. Scabies may also involve the face and head of babies.

Burrows are tortuous fine lines, often leading to a mite which may be removed with a needle for subsequent identification. Norwegian scabies is uncontrolled scabies in predisposed patients.

A scabies allergic rash may also be evident which is not immediately cured by treatment of the scabies: temporary antipruritic therapy is required such as crotamiton cream 10% or an oral antihistamine. The distribution of this rash does not correspond to the site of mite predilection. Animal scabies (including the 'mange' of dogs) can cause a papular irritant rash in contacts. The pets require treatment.

Therapy is usually with benzyl benzoate application BPC or γ-benzene hexachloride application.

(1) The patient has a hot bath at night and rubs his skin gently with a flannel.
(2) After drying with a towel, the application is painted on from the chin downwards to the soles of the feet.
(3) The skin is left unwashed for 24 hours, and the process repeated. All close contacts, especially sleeping partners, should be treated.

Other causes possibly associated with infection

Pemphigus vulgaris

This usually occurs after middle age and is a febrile bullous illness in which crops of blisters appear in the mouth or on the skin of the limbs and trunk. Lesions occur on pressure areas or areas that are traumatized. Nikolski's sign is positive – the superficial skin can be slid over deeper layers by lateral traction with a finger. The prognosis is poor, primarily because of secondary infections including a tendency to septicaemia.

173

Bullous pemphigoid

This usually occurs in old people. There are non-irritating tense blisters which may be several centimetres in diameter. The blisters tend not to be associated with separation of skin layers, and therefore Nikolski's sign is usually negative. Pemphigoid may be associated with underlying neoplasia and secondary infection is common.

Pityriasis rosea

This may commence abruptly and fever may be a feature: this rash consists of oval, brownish-red macules with their long axis along lines of natural skin cleavage. The edges of the lesions consist of a slight ridge of fine scales. Often a large 'herald' patch appears a few days before the main rash.

Polyarteritis nodosa

This may present with vasculitic lesions. There may be a fine netlike area of skin discolouration – livido reticularis. Arteritic skin infarction may occur as may frankly gangrenous areas. Arteries may be tender and nodular. The erythrocyte sedimentation rate is high and about 25–40% of patients are Australia antigen carriers.

Psoriasis

This is normally an afebrile condition consisting of well defined thickened red plaques with superficial silver scaling. It is often found on extensor surfaces and also on the elbows, knees and the scalp. 'Pseudo-infectious' presentations include acute guttate psoriasis, which may be precipitated by infection (particularly streptococcal sore throats) and acute pustular psoriasis which is a dermatological emergency.

Reiter's syndrome

Following an attack of non-specific urethritis or dysentery, a triad of urethritis, conjunctivitis and arthritis develops. Possible skin lesions include penile lesions (shallow erosions with a circinate outline) and keratoderma blenorrhagica (a pustular hyperkeratosis) which may affect the soles of the feet. Mouth ulcers are common.

OCCUPATIONAL INFECTIOUS DISEASES ASSOCIATED WITH RASHES

Anthrax

This is primarily a disease of those who come into contact with animal hides or certain other cattle-derived products.

Infection with *Bacillus anthracis* of the gut or lungs may occur, as may allergic lung disease. The cutaneous manifestation of skin-based infection is the malignant pustule which, curiously, is neither malignant nor pustular. The malignant pustule starts as a tiny papule crowned by a minute vesicle: this enlarges, becomes surrounded by a ring of vesicles, and the central area ulcerates forming a blackish depressed eschar. This eschar then spreads to cover the drying ring of vesicles. This lesion is usually non-painful – a point of diagnostic significance. Common sites include the forearm, head and neck. There is much soft tissue oedema.

Penicillin effects a bacteriological cure: alternatives are tetracyclines or erythromycin.

Brucellosis

Allergy to brucella antigens may give rise to transient maculopapular rashes shortly after exposure to the infected material.

Erysipelothrix insidiosa (rhusiopathiae)

This is usually a disease of those who handle dead animal tissue. Traumatic inoculation of the causative bacteria, usually into a finger, produces purplish-red inflammation. Usually there is no rapid spread, systemic upset or lymph node enlargement.

Orf (contagious ecthyma)

This is an uncommon disease caused by paravaccinia virus, and is usually acquired by those in contact with sheep or goats. The cutaneous lesion is initially an irritating maculopapular lesion followed by the development of a multiloculated vesicle which may evolve into a ragged superficial ulcer.

CUTANEOUS MANIFESTATIONS OF TROPICAL DISEASES

Patients with skin lesions who have been in the tropics or subtropics may have acquired an indigenous infection. The geographical distributions of major diseases that may be imported are detailed in Chapter 10. Although many diseases with cutaneous manifestations may be imported, the following diseases deserve special mention:

African viral haemorrhagic fevers

Marburg and Ebola virus infections are regularly associated with a maculo-papular rash with possible haemorrhagic elements: Lassa fever is occasionally associated with a rash.

175

Cutaneous larva migrans

Larvae of various hookworms (dog, cat and human) penetrate the skin (usually of the feet) and migrate 1–2 cm daily, giving rise to raised serpentine red lesions which are extremely irritant.

Cutaneous leishmaniasis

There is a wide spectrum of appearances and names (Aleppo boil, Delhi boil, Baghdad button, Oriental sore). Commonly there is a single lesion on the face or other exposed parts (where the sandfly has attacked). The lesions consist of a distinct circumscribed skin thickening with a 'miniodular' edge. Spontaneous healing would eventually occur leaving a depressed scar. The South American forms of cutaneous leishmaniasis are hardly ever imported.

Dengue

Various rashes may occur having macular, papular, reticular or petechial elements. There is fever and systemic upset including severe muscle and bone pains – 'breakbone fever'.

Jigger fleas (Tunga penetrans)

A female flea burrows into the skin to lay her eggs. Typically itchy or painful papule(s) occur on the lower limbs, often of those who have 'slept rough'.

Kala-azar

This gives rise to a generalized blackish cutaneous colouration which may be minimized if there is severe anaemia. Fever is present. Splenomegaly is usually well marked: lymph node enlargement and hepatomegaly are frequent.

Leprosy

Suspect leprosy if there are hypopigmented or erythematous skin areas which have impaired sensation with associated enlargement of local or other nerves. In addition to skin lesions there is often motor or sensory dysfunction of the peripheral nerves: the latter leads to painless burns or ulcers after minor trauma. Patients will probably have spent more than one year in the tropics or subtropics.

There is a spectrum of host responses to the leprosy bacillus.

In lepromatous leprosy (with little host resistance to invasion) there may be multiple symmetric papules or nodules anywhere on the body. Erythema nodosum leprosum may occur.

In tuberculoid leprosy the host resists the invading organism: usually there are only a few circular papules or plaques which are hairless, dry, relatively hypopigmented, have a raised edge, and the cutaneous sensation in the area of the lesion is reduced.

Intermediate forms of leprosy may occur. Depending on changes in host resistance skin lesions and peripheral nerves may become inflamed 'in reaction'.

The diagnosis of leprosy can be made clinically, and confirmed by smears of the exudate from skin slits stained for acid-fast bacilli. (*Myco. leprae* will not grow on inanimate media, unlike *Myco. tuberculosis.*)

Treatment should not be undertaken without consultation with an experienced specialist.

Loa loa

The adult worms may be noticed by the patient as they wriggle through the skin or eye. Five to ten centimetre diameter (Calabar) swellings can occur: each swelling lasts a few days and swellings are allergic reactions to the worms. There may be associated itching and urticaria.

Onchocerciasis

In established cases there may be fibrous skin nodules over bony prominences. Allergic reactions to the microfilaria produce persistent skin itching perhaps associated with an erythematous macular or papular rash with areas of altered skin pigmentation. Eosinophilia is present in all acute cases. Onchocerciasis may be confused with scabies.

Trypanosomiasis

A dusky red nodule (the chancre) at the site of the tsetse fly bite may be present on the patient or remembered. Within weeks of infection with *Trypanosoma rhodesiense* (or perhaps months in *Trypanosoma gambiense* infection) there is fever, headache and possibly a circinate erythematous rash. The rash lasts about 1 week and is readily seen in white skinned individuals. Always suspect trypanosomiasis in any patient from certain areas of Africa who develops personality or other cerebral changes.

Typhus fevers

These illnesses are usually transmitted by various insects including lice, fleas and mites.

In general, features of typhus fevers include an abrupt onset of fever with or without rigors, plus headache and constitutional upset. The rash usually develops about day 5 of illness, and initially consists of small maculopapular elements or purpuric lesions. In certain varieties of typhus, especially tick typhus, there may be an eschar – scab-like small (but diagnostically important) lesion where the infecting insect delivered the organisms.

In the absence of an eschar or a rash the differential diagnosis is very wide: after the emergence of the rash the important possibilities include meningococcal septicaemia, leptospirosis, a viral haemorrhagic fever, typhoid fever, salmonellosis, dengue, measles or rubella.

Confirmation of diagnosis is by testing for anti-Rickettsial antibodies using cross reacting strains of *Proteus* – the Weil-Felix reactions.

GENITAL MANIFESTATIONS OF SEXUALLY TRANSMITTED DISEASES

Patients with sexually transmitted diseases may present to Infectious Disease Units because the diagnosis of such a disease is uncertain, because the patient is systemically unwell, or because the referring doctor is horrified by the extent of the local lesions.

Ideally all patients with a sexually transmitted disease should be assessed at a special clinic, or subsequently referred for follow-up and initiation of contact tracing.

Urethritis

In the male the diagnosis of urethritis may be made by observing discharge (especially in the early morning pre-micturition state) or by the 'two glass test', in which a small quantity of urine is passed sequentially into two glasses. If both specimens are hazy there is phosphaturia or infection (not necessarily sexually transmitted infection) proximal to the anterior urethra. The urine is then acidified with acetic acid which will clear the opacity of phosphaturia: if there are hazy threads *in the first specimen only* there is anterior urethritis.

If gonorrhoea is suspected treatment should be given after appropriate specimens for microscopy, culture and sensitivity have been taken. As with all sexually transmitted diseases coincidental syphilis should be sought clinically and serologically.

Gonorrhoea

This is a highly infectious disease which may involve columnar or transitional epithelium of the urethra, rectum, pharynx and conjunctivae of both sexes, the endocervical canal in females or the vulva and vagina of prepubertal females.

In males the 'penile' symptoms are of pain or burning on micturition, and urethral discharge. Rectal symptoms may include discharge, tenesmus, bleeding, anal dampness, pruritis or discomfort. Epididymitis may occur.

In females genital gonorrhoea is often asymptomatic. 'Genital' symptoms include vaginal discharge, abnormal menstrual bleeding or anorectal discomfort. There may be labial pain from inflammation of Bartholins glands or lower abdominal pain from salpingitis. 'Urinary' symptoms include frequency or pain and burning on micturition.

Both sexes may have asymptomatic infection.

Standard treatment is with penicillins with or without probenecid, but penicillin resistance is often a problem and other drugs such as co-trimoxazole, kanamycin, spectinomycin, cephalosporins, tetracyclines and erythromycin have all been used. Unless follow-up can be guaranteed it seems sensible to utilize one dose therapy administered under supervision.

Non-specific urethritis

In patients with urethritis arising *de novo* or after gonococcal urethritis a cause may be demonstrated (including *Trichomonas*, *Candida*, *Chlamydia*, ureaplasma (a mycoplasma), urinary tract infection, herpes, warts or allergy to physical agents). However, in about 90% of patients investigated in a routine fashion there is no definitive diagnosis made, and the patient is then said to have non-specific urethritis.

Symptoms are commoner in males and are those of urethritis or urinary tract infection: occasionally a prostatitis may be associated. The urethral discharge contains white cells and is usually mucoid, but may be mucopurulent.

The diagnosis must only be made after the exclusion of the common pathogens. Gonorrhoea, in contrast to non-specific urethritis, is more severe and has a shorter incubation period. Non-specific urethritis occurring after an attack of gonorrhoea is referred to as post-gonococcal urethritis.

Treatment is with tetracyclines, the dosage and duration of which is debatable – usually for 2 weeks or more. Complications include prostatitis, epididymitis and Reiter's disease.

Balanitis

Balanitis (inflammation of the glans penis) or *posthitis* (inflammation of the underside of the prepuce).

These may have many causes including local trauma, mechanical irritants, poor personal hygiene, diabetes, antibacterial therapy, the

179

various infections detailed in this section or allergies (to rubber goods for example).

Clinically there is patchy erythema or superficial erosions on the relevant area: the presence of a white exudate suggests *Candida* infection whereas a thickish purulent exudate suggests *Trichomonas* infection.

Treatment is by encouraging personal hygiene and by treatment of the associated infection if any.

Syphilis

The characteristic manifestation of primary syphilis is the chancre which in males usually occurs on the penis, perianally or occasionally elsewhere. In females the chancre may occur on the genitalia or occasionally elsewhere. The chancre begins life as a small pink macule which becomes papular and then ulcerates: it is typically painless, non-tender and rounded, with a well defined margin and an indurated base. It does not bleed easily. Moderate regional lymph node enlargement is usual and typically the nodes are firm, discrete, painless, non-tender and unfixed to surrounding tissues.

Confirmation of the diagnosis is by darkground illumination of mobile treponemes obtained from a scrape of the chancre or by fluorescent antibody tests on this material. Serological tests for syphilis may be negative at this stage.

In secondary syphilis there may be local evidence of the more generalized rash, lymph node enlargement, mucosal lesions, or patches. Venereal warts may occurs in warm, moist areas, (such as the perineum—condylomata lata) and these are highly infectious.

Genital herpes infection

This is usually caused by type 2 herpes simplex infection. It presents as clusters of vesicles or pustules which may rupture to leave erosions. These lesions are usually rounded and superficial, they are painful or tender and may bleed when traumatized. Complicating secondary infection may arise. In the male lesions are mostly found on the glans, prepuce and shaft of the penis. The common sites in the female are the vulva or the cervix. Like type 1 herpes simplex infections recurrent attacks are not uncommon and frequently the first attack is the worst.

Treatment may be attempted with idoxuridine. Males should be advised to use a sheath for intercourse to prevent spread of infection.

Candida infection

This organism can be transmitted sexually. In the female there is a curd-like whitish discharge on a reddened mucosa with associated pruritis. If the discharge is profuse there may be pain or burning on micturition or dyspareunia. The urine should be tested for glucose. Treatment is with nystatin, amphotericin B, clotrimazole, miconazole or penotrane (hydrargaphen) pessaries.

Trichomonas vaginalis infection

In the symptomatic female there may be a profuse thin, yellow, frothy, malodorous vaginal discharge which causes vulval irritation or pain. In either sex there may be pain or burning on micturition and dyspareunia. In the male urethritis and irritation of the glans penis may result. The female: male ratio ratio of symptomatic cases is about 10 : 1. Diagnosis is confirmed by visualization or by culturing the causative protozoan. Treatment is usually with metronidazole for both the patient and the sexual partner(s).

Condyloma acuminata

These are papillomata. On cold dry areas these are small, flat areas resembling warts: in warm moist areas they are filiform and large. In the male they occur on the coronal sulcus of the penis, glans, frenum, the meatus, perianally and occasionally on the penile shaft. In the female the vulva, vagina and perianal area are commonly affected.

Treatment rests upon keeping the parts cool and dry if possible and topical application of podophyllin or trichloracetic acid. Occasionally cautery under general anaesthesia is necessary.

Obviously other more generalized skin conditions may affect the genitalia − particularly scabies or lice.

Chancroid (soft sore)

The major differentiating points from syphilis are in italics.

This highly infectious disease is found throughout the world but occurs more frequently in warm climates. A *painful* papule or vesicle rapidly progresses to form a pustule which then ulcerates: the ulcer *bleeds readily* and there is *no induration* (hence the name soft sore). The ulcer usually has a bright red overhanging edge and the ulcer base is a dirty, greyish-white exudate. In the male lesion(s) are usually on the penis and in the female there are usually multiple lesions around the clitoris and vulva.

Bubo formation may occur about 1−2 weeks after the local lesion or lesions: a mass of glands develops which may be *adherent to the skin* and which *may discharge*. There are often no systemic symptoms.

The diagnosis may be confirmed by identifying the causative agent, *Haemophilus ducreyi*, or by staining and culture of pus or material obtained from the ulcer surface.

181

Granuloma inguinale

This is usually a disease of tropical and subtropical areas and is a chronic slowly progressive ulcerative disease of the genitalia and adjacent tissues. Lesions are usually on the penile shaft, labia, perianal areas or intravaginally. Initially, a painless vesicle or indurated papule develops to form an ulcer 1–3 cm in diameter: this ulcer has a granular base and a rolled thickened edge.

Diagnosis is confirmed by microscopic identification of the diagnostic Donovan bodies in scrapings from the edge of an ulcer. The causative organism is *Donovania granulomatis (Calymmatobacterium granulomatis)*.

Lymphogranuloma venereum

This disease has a great prevalence in tropical and subtropical areas. In the primary stage there are small painless papule(s) or ulcers anywhere on the external genitalia but, unlike chancroid, these lesions only persist for a few days.

The disease's main effects result from damage to the lymphatic system draining the site of infection – a usual presentation is of unilateral or bilateral enlargement of inguinal nodes (bubos) occurring after the primary lesion has healed. In contrast to chancroid, lymphogranuloma venereum nodes are usually bilateral and fixed. Later lymphatic obstruction and fibrosis may occur with resultant anal strictures or vulval elephantiasis. A so-called genitoanorectal syndrome, perhaps with bloody mucopurulent rectal discharge, occurs in about 25% of patients in the late stage of this disease.

Diagnosis is confirmed by demonstrating or culturing the causative chlamydia in smears or aspirates of affected tissue: serological tests are available.

CUTANEOUS MANIFESTATIONS OF 'PARAINFECTIOUS' DISEASES

In my experience, these diseases may be referred initially to Infectious Diseases Units as 'fever plus a strange rash', as a 'pyrexial illness, ? cause', or as 'horrible spots? an infectious disease of some sort': indeed, some of these disorders may ultimately be found to have an infective causation.

Behçets syndrome

This may present as recurring episodes of oral and genital ulceration. It is a vasculitic syndrome of uncertain aetiology. Other manifestations include uveitis, central nervous system lesions, thrombophlebitis, erythema nodosum, arthritis or intestinal disease.

The genital ulcers are usually 5–20 mm in diameter, painful, have an erythematous halo (a diagnostically suggestive finding), and the base may have a yellow slough. In the male, the genital ulcers may be on the penis or scrotum, and in females on the labia.

Dermatitis herpetiformis

This usually occurs in association with gluten-sensitive enteropathy (which may be asymptomatic). There is an abrupt appearance of small patches of itchy vesicles with an erythematous base which, unlike herpes zoster, are not confined to dermatome distribution. All patients should be assessed for the presence of associated enteropathy (a gluten-free diet may cause the skin lesions to remit).

Dermatomyositis

Purplish discoloration of the face or eyelids occurs, perhaps with purple streaks on the dorsum of the fingers. The onset may be insidious or acute – the latter variety being admitted to Infectious Diseases Units as 'fever with a rash'. There may be muscle tenderness and weakness – particularly of proximal muscle groups.

Miliaria

These are small clear superficial vesicles often found on skin previously affected by sunburn. They are found on young children and other patients with high fevers, and they disappear rapidly on cooling. Milia rubra (prickly heat) often occurs in hot and humid conditions and is caused by sweat bursting out of blocked ducts and eliciting an inflammatory reaction which causes irritation (prickling) and itching.

DRUG ERUPTIONS

Drugs can cause almost any cutaneous eruption. Thus every patient with a rash should have a full pre-rash drug history elicited.

If an antibacterial drug had been given, decide for what reason it had been given: often it becomes apparent that children have been given antibacterial drugs for an unrecognized measles prodrome, or were given ampicillin or its derivatives for infectious mononucleosis.

The evolution of drug rashes may not conform to an infectious diseases rash of similar distribution – for example, measles evolves from above downwards.

Urticaria is suggestive of a drug allergy reaction, although occasionally an infection may be responsible. Eosinophilia also suggests a drug reaction, although certain infections, including scarlet fever, may be associated with an eosinophilia. (Table 11 details some common drug eruption patterns).

Table 11   Drug eruption patterns and some possible causes

Drug reaction pattern	*Some commonly used drugs that may be responsible*
Erythema nodosum	Oral contraceptives, sulphonamides
Exfoliative dermatitis	Penicillins, sulphonamides
Fixed drug eruptions – which recur at the same site each time the drug is taken	Tetracyclines, some laxatives
Measles-like (maculopapular)	Almost any drug, including antibacterial drugs and barbiturates
Mucocutaneous eruptions	Barbiturates, penicillins, sulphonamides, some antihypertensive and antidiabetic drugs
Photosensitive eruptions	Phenothiazines, sulphonamides, tetracyclines, thiazides
Purpuric eruptions	Anticoagulants, sulphonamides, thiazides
Toxic epidermal necrolysis	Barbiturates, penicillins, sulphonamides
Urticaria	Aspirin, penicillins, sulphonamides

Still's disease

Although also known as juvenile rheumatoid *arthritis*, a general systemic febrile disease without an obvious arthritic component may present as an infectious illness. Features include a high remittent fever, a characteristically flitting maculopapular rash which may appear and disappear repeatedly, lymph node enlargement, splenomegaly, hepatomegaly, pericarditis, weight loss and anaemia. A polymorphonuclear leukocytosis is common in the systemic form. The erythrocyte sedimentation is raised, which may be helpful in distinguishing this from the usual virus diseases of childhood in which the ESR is usually normal. The rheumatoid factor is present in about 10% of cases and the antinuclear factor present in about 30% of patients.

Systemic lupus erythematosus

There are skin manifestations in about 85% of patients with this 'autoimmune' disorder. Erythematous rashes are common and include the classical butterfly rash: Raynaud's syndrome is a common association. The ESR in systemic lupus erythematosus is usually very high; lupus erythematosus cell preparations are usually positive, as are tests for anti-nuclear and anti-DNA antibodies.

184

GLOSSARY OF DERMATOLOGICAL TERMS

ACNE: a specific skin disease with eruption of papules or pustules

ACUMINATE: sharp and pointed

BULLA: a blister – a localized collection of fluid in the epidermis usually more than 5 mm in diameter

CARBUNCLE: a necrotizing infection of skin and subcutaneous tissue with multiple formed or incipient drainage sinuses and an indurated border

CELLULITIS: inflammation of loose subcutaneous tissue

CHANCRE: the primary lesion of certain infections developing at the site of entry of the infection

CRUST: a formed outer layer of solid matter formed by drying of exudate or secretions

DISCRETE: made up of separated parts or characterized by lesions which do not become blended

ECCHYMOSIS: discoloration due to extravasation of blood

ENANTHEM: an eruption on a mucous surface – usually meaning oropharynx

ERYSIPELAS: a febrile illness characterized by inflammation and redness of the skin

ERYTHEMA: morbid redness of the skin due to congestion of the capillaries and which characteristically blanches on pressure

ERYTHRASMA: a chronic fungus infection of the skin with red or brownish patches usually on the side of the thighs, the scrotum or axilla

ESCHAR: a scab

EXANTHEM: an eruption or rash on the skin

FILARIFORM: threadlike

FOLLICULITIS: inflammation of excretory or secretory sacs or glands

FOMITES: any substance other than food that may harbour or transmit infectious organisms

FURUNCLE: a boil. A painful nodule in the skin with circumscribed inflammation

GUTTATE: resembling a drop

HERPETIFORM: characterized by clusters of small vesicles

INDOLENT: causing little or no pain

INFESTATION: establishment of organisms of the phyllum Arthropoda upon or within the body of the host

INFECTION: a morbid state caused by multiplication of pathogenic microorganisms within the body

INTERTRIGO: a chafed patch of skin especially on opposed surfaces

LICHENIFIED: thickened and hardened skin

LUPUS: having an appearance like a wolf

MACULE: a small discoloured circumscribed superficial non-elevated area of skin

NODULE: a palpable solid or round lesion deeper in the skin than a papule

PAPILLOMA: an epithelial tumour in which cells cover finger-like processes or ridges of stroma

PAPULE: a small superficial circumscribed solid elevation of the skin usually less than 1 cm in diameter

PARONYCHIA: inflammation involving the folds of tissue surrounding the fingernail

PETECHIAE: small spots formed by effusion of blood

PLAQUE: an elevated patch or flat area more than 1 cm in diameter

PLEOMORPHIC: occurring in various distinct forms

POCK: a pustule

POX: an eruptive disease

PURPURA: a condition characterized by petechiae or confluent ecchymoses

PUS: liquid inflammatory products made up of cells (leukocytes) and thin fluid

PUSTULE: a small elevation of the skin filled with pus

RETICULAR: resembling a network

SQUAMOUS: scaly or plate-like patches

SUPPURATION: the formation of pus

SYMMETRICAL: regular distribution around a common axis – usually around the midline

URTICARIA: a vascular reaction pattern marked by transient, smooth, slightly elevated patches which are redder or paler than surrounding skin. It is usually itchy

VERRUCA: a wart

VESICLE: an elevated skin lesion up to 5 mm in diameter containing fluid

VITILIGO: smooth light coloured patches

WHEAL: a transient circumscribed red-white elevation of the skin 0.5–10 cm in diameter caused by local oedema

Suggested further reading

Emond, R.T.D. (1974). *A Colour Atlas of Infectious Diseases*. (London: Wolfe Medical Publications)

Peters, W. and Gilles, H.M. (1977). *A Colour Atlas of Tropical Medicine and Parasitology*. (London: Wolfe Medical Publications)

Wisdom, A. (1973). *A Colour Atlas of Venereology*. (London: Wolfe Medical Publications)

12
Infection-related diseases of the nervous system

Nervous system dysfunction may be diffuse or localized, and localizing signs (Table 12) should be sought in all patients with suspected nervous system infection. There are several sites at which the nervous system can be affected by infection (Figure 43). In acute infections affecting the central nervous system (CNS) there may be suggestive signs of meningitis (inflammation of the lining membranes of the brain) or of encephalitis (inflammation of brain substance (Table 13), although abscess formation may occasionally present as a space occupying lesion with no features to suggest an infection-related aetiology. The differential diagnosis of disorders which cause diffuse dysfunction of the CNS are listed in Table 14. For the purpose of this chapter, the *central nervous system* refers to structures of the brain and spinal cord, except the anterior horn (motor) cells, and the *peripheral nervous system* refers to the peripheral nerve fibres outside the brain and spinal cord but including the anterior horn cells within the spinal cord.

The lumbar puncture results are of such crucial diagnostic, therapeutic and prognostic importance that it is fully justified to classify nervous system infections according to the CSF findings. In practice a useful differentiation can be made between CNS infections which are associated

187

Table 12   Possible clinical signs associated with localized nervous system lesions

Upper motor neurone lesions
Clonus present
Abdominal reflexes absent unilaterally
Weakness
Spasticity
Tendon reflexes increased
'Clasp-knife' phenomenon present
Increased tone in antigravity muscles
(Initially a flaccid paralysis may be present as in spinal shock and later signs may include contractures and trophic changes)

Lower motor neurone lesions
Flaccid paralysis
Absent reflexes
Fasciculation
(Later signs include contractures and trophic changes)

Dominant hemisphere lesions
Hemiplegia
Focal or generalized seizures
Dysphasia − expressive (motor)
        − receptive (sensory)
Dyslexia
Dysgraphia
Dyscalculia
Apraxia
Agnosia (failure of recognition)

Non-dominant hemisphere lesions
Hemiplegia
Visiospatial impairment
Focal or generalized seizures

Cerebellar lesions
Intention tremor
Scanning speech   } Charcot's triad
Nystagmus
Hypotonia
Pendular tendon reflexes
Abnormalities of co-ordination including: typical gait, dysmetria, dyssynergia.

Bulbar palsy (a bilateral lower motor neurone lesion involving the lower cranial nerves)

Dysarthria
Dysphagia
A weak wasted tongue
Fasciculation of tongue

Pseudobulbar palsy (a bilateral upper motor neurone lesion)
Spasticity
Hyper-reflexia
Extensor plantar responses
Dysarthria
Dysphagia
Inappropriate emotional responses
(Rarely myositis causes weakness of the bulbar muscles)

Brain stem lesions
Nystagmus
Vomiting
Increased muscle tone
Hyper-reflexia
Opisthotonus
Extension of limbs
Hyperpyrexia
Sweating
Horner's syndrome
Rapid respiration
Tachycardia
'Crossed' cranial nerve palsies

Basal ganglia lesions (including Parkinson's disease, Wilson's disease and phenothiazine overdosage)
Bradykinesia
Cogwheel rigidity
Tremor
Positive glabellar tap

Tentorial herniation
Initially a unilaterally dilating pupil
Third nerve external ophthalmoplegia
Deteriorating conscious level
With a supratentorial lesion ipsilateral hemiplegia may occur as the opposite cerebral peduncle is compressed against the tentorial edge
Quadriplegia with decerebrate posture.

with a pyogenic CSF (pyogenic = having a raised CSF polymorphonuclear white cell count) and infections associated with a lymphocytic CSF. In the former, 'instant' lumbar puncture, blood cultures, identification and treat-

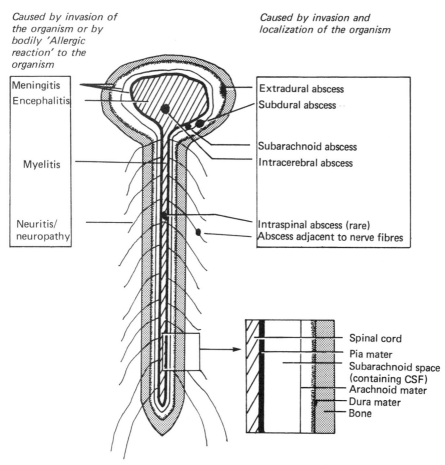

Caused by invasion of the organism or by bodily 'Allergic reaction' to the organism

Caused by invasion and localization of the organism

Meningitis
Encephalitis

Myelitis

Neuritis/neuropathy

Extradural abscess
Subdural abscess

Subarachnoid abscess
Intracerebral abscess

Intraspinal abscess (rare)
Abscess adjacent to nerve fibres

Spinal cord
Pia mater
Subarachnoid space (containing CSF)
Arachnoid mater
Dura mater
Bone

Figure 43   The possible sites of nervous system dysfunction caused by infection or infectious diseases. (Schematic section through brain and spinal cord)

Table 13   Possible symptoms and signs associated with meningitis and encephalitis

Meningitis	*Encephalitis*
Headache	Possibly meningitic signs
Neck stiffness	Impaired conscious level
Positive Kernig's sign (spasm of the hamstrings when the knee is extended after the hip is fully flexed)	Abnormal mentation
	Abnormal behaviour
	Drowsiness leading to coma
	Focal neurological signs
	Epileptic seizures

Common to both
Fever
Raised intracranial pressure
(CSF pressure high)

ment of the causative organism are mandatory, whilst infections associated with a lymphocytic CSF in general usually do not require such urgent confirmation. (Tuberculous meningitis is one exception to this generalization.) The classical CSF findings in various infections of the CNS are given in Tables 39 and 40 in Chapter 15.

If there is a suspicion of a meningitis, the peripheral blood count is of secondary interest to the differential CSF cell count.

Table 14 The differential diagnosis of disease causing diffuse dysfunction of the central nervous system

Cerebral malaria
Demyelination (especially in the brain stem)
Disseminated intravascular coagulation
Encephalitis/encephalomyelitis
Head injury
Meningitis
Metabolic dysfunctions (including drug overdoses)
Multiple microemboli (e.g. fat emboli)
Pituitary infarction
Post-ictal states
Rising intracranial pressure (with coning)
Septicaemia
Subarachnoid haemorrhage

The following two features are useful but occasionally fallible generalizations:

(1) In established pyogenic meningitis the patient's conscious level is usually impaired. In lymphocytic meningitis the patient may have a severe headache but, in the absence of tuberculous meningitis, usually has an unimpaired conscious level and can give a lucid history. In conditions as serious as meningitis, clinical impressions should not be trusted and a lumbar puncture (LP) should be performed on most patients in whom meningitis is a possibility: one possible exception is classical mumps with a confirmatory serum amylase elevation.

(2) Patients with meningism and a purpuric rash most likely have a meningococcal septicaemia with either active or impending meningitis and should be treated for meningococcal infection even if the CSF results are normal.

Problems arise

(1) When patients with pyogenic meningitis present early in the course of their illness and when their conscious level may not be

impaired. Prior ineffective antibacterial therapy may partially or completely suppress both the symptoms and the signs of meningitis.

Prior antibacterial therapy reduces the chances of bacterial identification on CSF Gram stain, and on CSF and blood culture. However, it is unusual for prior therapy to change a pyogenic (polymorphonuclear) CSF into a totally lymphocytic CSF. In general, if the CSF contains more than 1200 cells per cubic mm, more than 0.8 g/litre protein and less than 2.5 mmol/litre of glucose then pyogenic meningitis is almost certain.

Occasionally prior antibacterial therapy may abolish these findings so that a pyogenic meningitis produces a predominantly lymphocytic CSF (suggestive of viral meningitis) but in this case the CSF glucose is usually lower than occurs in classical viral meningitis. In these circumstances, the differential diagnosis would lie between partially treated pyogenic meningitis and tuberculous meningitis: differentiation may be problematical as tubercle bacilli are notoriously difficult to visualize in the CSF.

(2)　When there are no signs to suggest the presence of underlying CNS infection. This may occur in neonates, the elderly, the very ill, unconscious patients or in the preterminal stages of meningitis.

(3)　When the CSF microscopy results are equivocal. In these circumstances further urgent investigations may be of assistance, but pending results treatment should often be started on a best 'informed guess' basis.

The majority of the possible organisms responsible for CNS infections are listed in Figure 44, and the following account deals with these in sequence.

PYOGENIC MENINGITIS: THE THREE COMMON PATHOGENS

Pyogenic meningitis is an acute medical emergency. Any patient with a brief febrile illness with headache, fever, impaired mental function and signs of meningitis should have his CSF examined without delay. In almost all cases of pyogenic meningitis the CSF will be under increased pressure, be cloudy or purulent, have a raised polymorphonuclear leukocyte count, have a low glucose level and a raised protein level. The organism responsible, even if not seen on Gram's stain, is usually grown in culture; if a patient has an acute pyogenic meningitis and no organisms are visualized or grown, the most likely organism responsible is the meningococcus.

In every case of pyogenic meningitis, therapy should be commenced as soon as the CSF and blood cultures have been obtained: modification of initial therapy can be made when the results of Gram's stain and later culture are available.

In Britain, the 'big three' organisms responsible for bacterial meningitis are *Haemophilus influenzae, Neisseria meningitidis* and *Strep. pneumoniae.*

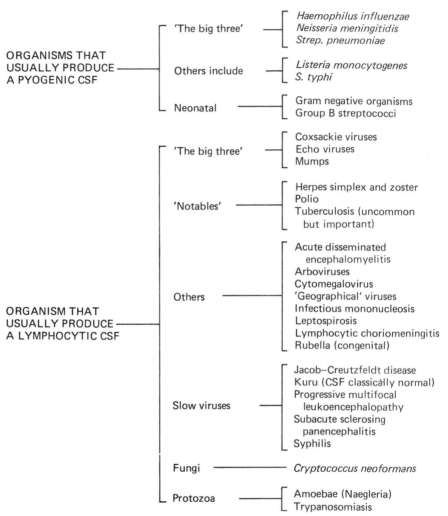

Figure 44   Organisms that infect the CNS and which may cause a pyogenic or lymphocytic CSF

Haemophilus influenzae

Haemophilus influenzae meningitis is predominantly a disease of the under-fives and classically presents with a picture of relatively slow onset pyogenic meningitis without a rash: it may occasionally present with signs related more to complications (such as sub-dural effusions) rather than a meningitis. Treatment is with chloramphenicol or high dose ampicillin but as there are ampicillin resistant strains chloramphenicol is usually favoured.

Meningococcal meningitis

Meningococcal meningitis can affect any age but is more common in the young. It can cause death within hours despite appropriate therapy and thus early diagnosis and treatment are essential. It may present as a meningitic illness, a septicaemic illness or both. The major clue to the meningococcal aetiology is the presence of a purpuric rash which is present in at least a third of patients with meningitis. The assoc-iated septicaemia may cause septicaemic shock, circulatory failure and disseminated intravascular coagulation (including the Waterhouse–Friderickson syndrome). Relatively minor complications such as pericard-itis, polyarthritis and pleurisy may occur. The CSF findings are usually typical of an acute pyogenic meningitis, with gram-negative diplococci being seen intracellularly in polymorphonuclear cells.

Treatment is usually with high dose penicillin intravenously (to ensure delivery to the brain and to avoid painful injections) possibly including sulphonamides. (Sulphonamides are not used alone because resistant strains are common.) Chloramphenicol, although bacteriostatic, is probably the drug of second choice: it is bacteriologically appropriate and penetrates well into the CNS. Septicaemic shock with hypotension may need to be treated in its own right, and the patient if comatose should be nursed appropriately.

Close contacts of a case should be given prophylaxis *as soon as is possible*. Penicillin is *not* appropriate for prophylaxis as it does not clear meningococcal bacteria from the throat, possibly because it does not penetrate well into the secretions of the uninflamed throat. Sulphon-amides, rifampicin or minocycline are appropriate drugs for prophylaxis and often the choice depends on the sensitivities of current local strains.

Pneumococcal meningitis

Often there is an underlying cause for infection with this organism, possibly a respiratory tract infection (lungs, sinuses or ears), a history of past or present head injury with or without a known skull fracture (all patients with meningitis should have their skull palpated for the presence of fractures or to detect tenderness related to sinusitis or mastoiditis), or an underlying predisposition to pneumococcal infection such as alcoholism or splenectomy. There is no rash.

Treatment is with high dosage penicillin to which, in the United Kingdom, the pneumococcus is almost invariably sensitive.

OTHER CAUSES OF PYOGENIC MENINGITIS

Listeria meningitis

This may occur in neonates who acquire infection from the maternal birth canal. It may also occur in older people secondary to septicaemia. It presents as a pyogenic meningitis but the organism can often be dismissed as a 'contaminating diphtheroid'. It is sensitive to a wide range of antibacterial drugs.

Moraxella/acinobacter (Mima polymorphea)

This organism may produce an illness complete with rash, which is similar to meningococcal meningitis but it is not sensitive to penicillin: tetracyclines or kanamycin are possible therapies.

Typhoid fever

Although mental symptoms and headache are common, true meningitis is uncommon. Meningitis when it does occur is pyogenic in nature and carries an extremely grave prognosis.

Other organisms which may cause bacterial meningitis include staphylococci, group A streptococci and *Pseudomonas*.

NEONATAL MENINGITIS

Neonatal meningitis is a serious disease and early diagnosis is of paramount importance. The slightest suspicion of meningitis in an ill neonate requires its exclusion. The early signs may be non-specific (Table 15); the only clue may be the presence of a bulging anterior fontanelle, but even this may be absent if there is associated severe dehydration. Thus it is not surprising that neonatal meningitis is a disease of high morbidity and mortality: the death rate can approach 60% and up to 40% of the survivors show signs of physical or intellectual damage.

Table 15   The approximate incidence of signs in neonatal meningitis: note the rarity of neck stiffness

Fever	60%	Irritability	30%
Lethargy	50%	Jaundice	30%
Anorexia/vomiting	50%	Bulging fontanelle	30%
Respiratory distress	50%	Diarrhoea	20%
Convulsions	40%	Neck stiffness	15%

Particularly at risk are neonates with spina bifida and other congenital deformities of the CNS, premature babies, and neonates born to mothers who experienced delay between rupture of the membranes and delivery. In most studies of neonatal meningitis, gram negative bacteria (particularly *E. coli*) predominate as causative organisms along with group B streptococci.

Drugs useful in therapy include gentamicin alone or in various combinations, chloramphenicol and co-trimoxazole. Gentamicin has a broad spectrum of activity including gram negative enterobacteria and *Pseudomonas*, but streptococci are usually resistant and, in addition, a penicillin may be indicated. However there are problems in relation to gentamicin therapy in that CSF penetration is poor: ideally gentamicin should be given by the intrathecal route − but even this route does not guarantee adequate ventricular drug levels and many authorities would recommend insertion of a ventricular catheter for therapy. Chloramphenicol has a broad spectrum of activity (excluding *Pseudomonas*) and CSF penetration is very satisfactory without the need to utilize the intrathecal route. Co-trimoxazole is favoured in some units but again *Pseudomonas* is notably resistant.

Whichever drugs are used appropriate levels should be checked to ensure effective concentrations are being achieved. Routine administration of anticonvulsants and steroids have also been advocated, but such therapies are controversial.

Complications of neonatal meningitis may occur even after seemingly adequate therapy and include persistent inflammation of the ventricles (ventriculitis), subdural effusions and hydrocephalus due to blockage of CSF drainage routes (monitor head circumference during and after treatment). Later complications include deafness, cerebral palsy and epilepsy.

LYMPHOCYTIC MENINGITIS: THE THREE COMMON PATHOGENS

Lymphocytic meningitis is usually caused by non-bacterial agents although several bacteria (including spirochaetes and mycobacteria) are classically associated with a lymphocytic CSF. An additional difficulty is that CSF obtained *early* in the course of a lymphocytic meningitis may show a predominantly polymorphonuclear response, but in this case the *total* cell count is usually low and less than would be expected in a pyogenic meningitis. If the CSF cell count is equivocal and other tests (see Chapter 15) are not of help a repeat lumbar puncture should be considered as this may reveal diagnostic trends in various CSF parameters.

In Britain today the 'big three' causes of lymphocytic meningitis are coxsackie, Echo and mumps viruses.

Coxsackie and Echo virus meningitis

These are both enteroviruses and may or may not cause gastrointestinal symptoms in relation to a meningitis. Each may produce a rash which may resemble meningococcal purpura. Manifestations peripheral to the CNS, such as herpangina or Bornholm disease, may also provide an aetiological clue to infection with these viruses. These viruses may be cultured from the throat or stool but confirmation that the virus was pathogenic also requires a more than fourfold change in serum antibody levels. Isolation of a particular virus *from the CSF* is sufficient in itself to label that virus as pathogenically significant.

Mumps meningitis

This may or may not be associated with other manifestations of mumps. A raised serum amylase level is circumstantial diagnostic evidence only, as other organisms may occasionally produce a pancreatitis or parotitis associated with a meningitis.

OTHER CAUSES OF LYMPHOCYTIC MENINGITIS

Herpes simplex

This may cause a meningitis which has a curious predilection for the temporal lobes where it may cause an associated encephalitis with mental, behavioural and memory abnormalities: epileptic seizures and focal neurological signs may also occur.

Herpes simplex is probably the commonest cause of sporadic severe encephalitis: it can affect any age but the majority of reported cases occur in the first year of life, often in the first month. Herpetic lesions are present on the skin or in the mouth to give a diagnostic clue in only a small proportion of sufferers; even this clue may be misleading because herpes febrilis can be an incidental finding in many infections. Treatment of progressive herpes simplex encephalitis is with adenine arabinoside but the overall prognosis is very poor once focal neurological signs or coma develop.

Herpes virus varicella–zoster

Infections may be associated with a mild self-limiting encephalitis which may cause cerebellar dysfunction of which nystagmus is frequently the only sign. Rarely adenine arabinoside may be required.

Poliomyelitis

In Britain, polio is an uncommon disease, largely due to the effectiveness of vaccination. In those infected, clinical features may be absent or so vague as to be undiagnosable (abortive polio) but a proportion of infected patients will progress and develop 'minor' symptoms and, after a possible brief respite, a paralytic 'major' illness may develop. In the pre-paralytic phase it is impossible to deduce with certainty the causative virus, although certain epidemiological features may be suggestive. There may be marked muscle pains which may be suggestive of polio, although other infections, especially leptospirosis, can cause pain. There are usually no sensory *signs*.

The paralytic stage of illness is often preceded by muscular fasciculation but sphincter disturbance is rare. In common with other causes of lower motor neurone paralysis, there is loss of power, wasting of affected muscles and loss of associated reflexes. (Secondary orthopaedic complications may follow this loss of muscle power.) It is essential to distinguish between pharyngeal paralysis with accumulation of saliva in the pharynx and paralysis of respiratory muscles: both can present with respiratory embarrassment and be fatal, but treatment of each is obviously different. Usually most of the paralysis occurs in the first 24 hours after onset of paralysis but progression may occur for about 3 days or until the fever remits. The extent of paralysis is variable and appears to bear some relation to the use of muscle groups during the pre-paralytic stage. Recovery is essentially unpredictable, some anterior horn cells appear to sustain only temporary damage and recovery commences within the first week, but if muscles are still paralysed at the end of a month they are likely to remain paralysed, although late recovery may still occur in the neck muscles, the diaphragm and muscles supplied by the cranial nerves.

In a pre-paralytic illness with signs of meningeal irritation, the CSF becomes progressively lymphocytic, although in the early stages a low cell count may contain up to about 50% of polymorphonuclear cells: paralytic polio is almost invariably associated with a lymphocytic pleocytosis.

The differential diagnosis of polio

Even the paralytic stage is not specific to polio as the other enteroviruses (coxsackie and Echo viruses) may produce a similar pattern of paralysis, but with a better prognosis in terms of eventual recovery.

In the pre-paralytic stage of polio limb tenderness and pain may be confused with osteomyelitis, pyogenic arthritis, myositis or leptospirosis. Other conditions which may cause confusion include *transverse myelitis*, in which flaccid paralysis is associated with extensor plantar responses, sensory signs and loss of sphincter control. *Encephalomyelitis* (which may complicate infectious illnesses or immunizations) is usually obvious from the case history and also both motor and sensory tracts may be involved. In polio paralysis is usually asymmetrical and patchy (unlike that found in Guillain–Barré syndrome or botulism).

Occasionally diagnostic confusion may result if a vaccine strain of polio virus is isolated from a patient with an illness unrelated to polio but which has CNS features. Even more confusingly it is possible that vaccine strains may cause a CNS illness including paralysis but this is very rare.

Principles of treatment of polio

Absolute rest is essential in the paralytic stage and even before this if polio is anticipated. Paralysed limbs are kept in position with sandbags and pillows. During convalescence, passive movements should be performed along with appropriate splinting so that contractures do not occur. Galvanic stimulation of denervated muscles is useful. Respiratory paralysis may require appropriate measures including ventilation. Respiratory function should be measured by spirometer (not shared with other patients) or less accurately by serial monitoring of the maximum figure attained in progressive counting in one expiration.

Tuberculous meningitis

This can occur in any age group, but is most common in young children. The onset of specifically meningitic symptoms and signs is usually insidious with vague prodromal ill health comprising malaise, apathy and anorexia rather than headache, vomiting, fever, neck stiffness and impairment of consciousness. However tuberculous meningitis may present clinically as an acute meningitis and even a CSF polymorphonuclear leukocytosis of 15 000–23 000 could be compatible with a diagnosis of tuberculous meningitis.

Cranial nerve paralysis may occur because of cranial nerve fibre damage or because of involvement of nervous tissue by arteritis. Signs of widespread CNS involvement may become evident: these are caused by arteritis, ischaemia, infarction, oedema, immune reactions or glial reactions, often resulting in limb paralysis. Retinal choroid tubercles are visible on ophthalmoscopy in about 25% of patients with miliary tuberculosis and are diagnostic of tuberculosis: they are round or oval yellowish lesions about half the size of the optic disc. Phlyctenular conjunctivitis can occur as an allergic reaction to any protein substance but most instances are caused by tuberculo-protein hypersensitivity: they are pinkish-yellow spots in the conjunctival epithelium, limbus or cornea. With the exception of the cornea there is surrounding vascular engorgement.

Cerebral tuberculosis may rarely manifest as a solitary localized granulomatous mass (a tuberculoma) which presents as a space occupying lesion or, if leakage occurs into the CSF, as an associated tuberculous meningitis. A frequent clue to the presence of this organism is evidence of tuberculous infection elsewhere (which presumably initiated spread to the CNS): the chest X-ray may reveal active tuberculosis, either of primary or secondary complex pattern with possible evidence of miliary spread. The Mantoux test is positive in about 80% of cases but may be negative particularly if the patient is ill with an overwhelming tuberculosis. The CSF is usually under increased pressure, often clear or slightly turbid, a fine cobweb clot may form on standing, and there is usually a lymphocytic pleocytosis although in the early stages polymorphonuclear cells may predominate. The host's immune reactions play a major pathogenic role: the organisms are scanty and if these are not detected there may be diagnostic confusion with viral meningitis, as both tuberculous and viral meningitis produce a lymphocytic CSF. However the glucose level in tuberculous meningitis is characteristically low and the protein level is often raised. If these findings occur and no malignant cells are seen in a centrifuged deposit of CSF, it may well be sensible to treat for tuberculous meningitis pending further elucidation.

Treatment

Therapy of tuberculous meningitis is somewhat controversial as controlled trials are difficult to perform in this relatively uncommon disease. The general principles of antituberculous therapy as outlined in Chapter 2 are applicable. Initial treatment is usually with at least three standard first-line antituberculous drugs, remembering that certain of these drugs do not cross the blood–brain barrier in adequate concentrations, and it may be necessary to give them intrathecally. Isoniazid, pyrazinamide and ethionamide penetrate the CSF satisfactorily but streptomycin and ethambutol only penetrate well if the meninges are inflamed. Rifampicin penetrates the CSF poorly – but poor penetration of a drug highly effective against tuberculosis does not imply lack of useful activity in the concentrations actually achieved in the CSF. Streptomycin and isoniazid can, if necessary, be given intrathecally by the lumbar route although this route does not guarantee adequate intraventricular levels.

Routine administration of steroids is controversial: most doctors would only use these for impending or proven blockage of CSF pathways.

UNCOMMON INFECTIVE CAUSES OF A LYMPHOCYTIC MENINGITIS

Arboviruses

Arboviruses are important tropical and subtropical causes of meningitis and encephalitis. The only arbovirus infection endemic in Britain is

Louping ill, an encephalitic disease of man transferred from sheep by ticks: it is an occupational risk for shepherds in Scotland.

Acute disseminated (post-infectious) encephalomyelitis

This is a syndrome that may occur shortly after a variety of infections including measles, rubella, vaccinia and chickenpox. The means by which damage is caused are uncertain – 'allergic' is as good a label as any. Neurological signs relate to the site and extent of nervous system damage. The onset is usually rapid and clinical signs range from trivial irritability or drowsiness to coma and death. Signs of meningeal or cerebral irritation are frequent and may be followed by convulsions and coma. The CSF may be normal but is usually lymphocytic, with an increase in the protein level. The prognosis is often uncertain in the acute stage and treatment is essentially supportive. Steroids have been advocated but their role is uncertain.

Cytomegalovirus (CMV)

Cytomegalovirus (CMV) may cause a congenital or acquired meningo-encephalitis. Congenital CMV infection of a child *in utero* usually occurs during an initial infection of the mother. Possible manifestations of congenital CMV infection other than meningoencephalitis include microcephaly, hepatosplenomegaly, jaundice, purpura, mental retardation, spasticity, epilepsy, visual defects or cerebral calcification. The overall prognosis is poor. The differential diagnosis includes congenital rubella (in which cataract, deafness and congenital heart lesions may be present), neonatal sepsis, generalized herpes simplex infection and congenital toxoplasmosis (which may be seen in an appropriately stained CSF deposit – but often differentiation depends on serological tests). Choroidoretinitis may occur in congenital CMV infection: however it may also occur in congenital rubella and toxoplasmosis. The finding of choroidoretinitis would (statistically) favour a diagnosis of toxoplasmosis.

'Geographical viruses'

Geographical viruses (often arboviruses) are those with a limited geographical distribution and indeed often have a place or area title.

Infectious mononucleosis

This may produce a mild meningitic or encephalitic illness: both are uncommon.

Leptospirosis

Infection with *L. icterohaemorrhagica* is commonly an occupation-related disease in those exposed to the urine of rats (sewer workers, farm workers and fishyard workers). Infection with *L. canicola* is often acquired from the urine of dogs – a historical point not to be forgotten in a patient with a lymphocytic meningitis of uncertain aetiology. Many other strains of leptospires can initiate a meningitis.

Other characteristic symptoms of leptospirosis may be present to give diagnostic clues but a meningitis can be the only sign of leptospirosis. The diagnosis is simple if there is a full-blown Weil's syndrome with jaundice, renal impairment, conjunctival injection, a high white cell count in the blood and a raised erythrocyte sedimentation rate. In established cases with meningitic involvement there is a lymphocytic CSF although polymorphs may predominate early in the course of meningeal irritation. The meningitis itself is rarely a life-threatening disease. Diagnosis is by demonstration of the organism on dark ground microscopy of CSF or urine and by appropriate serology. Treatment is supportive with either penicillin or a tetracycline as antibacterial therapy.

Lymphocytic choriomeningitis

This is a self-limiting meningitis usually lasting 7–10 days. It is a disease usually acquired from mice and the pathogenesis depends on the host's immunological (predominantly lymphocytic) reaction to the virus.

Rubella

Congenital rubella may manifest with eye, heart or ear damage. There may be purpura, anaemia, thrombocytopenia, bone changes or jaundice. The CSF is frequently abnormal with increase in cells or protein or both.

Syphilis

A lymphocytic meningitis may occur in secondary syphilis and the classical copper-coloured non-itchy rash may provide a clue. Any non-meningococcal lymphocytic meningitis with a rash that occurs in known or suspected homosexuals should be strongly suspected as having a syphilitic aetiology and the appropriate studies performed on serum and CSF. In about 10% of untreated patients with secondary syphilis neurological and other tertiary manifestations may present years after the primary infection.

Neurological manifestations of tertiary syphilis may be caused by gumma formation, meningovascular syphilis, a parenchymatous syphilis or tabes dorsalis.

Gummas

These are large granulomas characterized by extensive caseation necrosis that can occur anywhere in the nervous system and present with signs related to a space occupying lesion.

Meningovascular syphilis

This infection leads to meningeal thickening with cranial nerve palsies, Argyll Robertson pupils (small, irregular pupils which react to accommodation but not to light), or strokes and signs of ischaemia caused by an endarteritis obliterans.

Parenchymatous syphilis

In this the parenchyma of the brain and spinal cord are damaged leading to general paralysis of the insane, epilepsy, possibly Argyll Robertson pupils, tremor (often marked in the facial muscles and tongue), slow slurred speech, and progressive neurological deterioration with mental changes. The plantar responses are extensor and tendon reflexes increased unless spinal changes interrupt the reflex arcs. In general paralysis of the insane the cerebral cortex is damaged: sensation is usually intact unless spinal damage is present.

Tabes dorsalis (locomotor ataxia)

There are degenerative changes in the posterior columns and root ganglia of the spinal cord. Symptoms include sensory loss, analgesia, impairment of postural sensation, impairment of vibration sensation and deficient muscle stretch sensation, all of which contribute to ataxia which often is worse in the dark (as vision cannot then compensate for these deficiencies). Dorsal root damage may be associated with lightning pains (brief paroxysms of stabbing pains) and there may be sexual and excretory malfunctions due to loss of sensory innervation.

Treatment of syphilis is with penicillin, although this obviously cannot reverse severe damage sustained in tertiary syphilis. Erythromycin and tetracyclines are alternatives. *Treponema pallidum* is not sensitive to co-trimoxazole. Within 6–12 hours of the administration of penicillin, a (Jarish–Herxheimer) reaction may occur with transient fever, malaise, headache, myalgia and exacerbation of focal lesions. Bed rest and analgesia may suffice but prophylactic steroids are sometimes used to abort this reaction.

Fungal causes of lymphocytic meningitis

Cryptococcus neoformans

This organism is also known as *Torula histolytica* and the disease as Torulosis. Infection is usually metastatic from the lungs and an irregular, granulomatous thickening of the meninges occurs. Infection with this organism should be suspected in the immunosuppressed, those with lymphomas, leukaemias and other malignancies. Clinically there is an insidious onset of symptoms and signs. Although meningitic signs are usually present, focal CNS damage and papilloedema may occur in the absence of meningitic signs and thus might be misleadingly suggestive of cerebral tumour or secondary deposits. The CSF findings are variable ranging from a clear fluid with a small excess of cells and protein to a (usually lymphocytic) pleocytosis with or without a high protein content. The differential diagnosis lies between other subacute or chronic meningitides (including tuberculosis), sarcoidosis or intracranial tumour. The diagnosis will often be missed unless the CSF is specifically stained and cultured for fungi. Treatment is with amphotericin B, 5-fluorocytosine or a combination of the two drugs.

Aspergillus, candida and histoplasma are other fungi which may cause a meningitis.

Protozoan causes of lymphocytic meningoencephalitis

Trypanosomiasis

Although acute onset rapidly progressive CNS disturbance may occur in *T. rhodesiense* infection there is usually a chronic fluctuating illness with progressive apathy, drowsiness, dysarthria and involuntary movements. It must be suspected in patients who have been in certain areas of Equatorial Africa within the previous few years and who have marked personality change or other cerebral symptoms.

Diagnosis is by demonstration of the organism in the peripheral blood or in lymph node aspirate. Serological tests are available and characteristically the serum IgM is raised.

Other protozoa that can cause a meningitis or encephalitic picture include amoebae and toxoplasmosis.

The differential diagnoses of lymphocytic meningitis are listed in Table 17.

Treatment of viral meningitis and encephalitis

Most patients with acute viral *meningitis* make a spontaneous recovery and treatment is largely symptomatic, including adequate analgesia.

Patients with a treatable viral *encephalitis* may require treatment if their condition is desperate or deteriorating. Relatively non-specific treatments which may be used include steroids and ACTH which are probably beneficial by reducing raised intracranial pressure caused by oedema, thereby 'buying time' for the host's defences to deal with the infection. Relief of raised intracranial pressure may be achieved by other means, including infusions of mannitol, hypothermia, hyperventilation or surgical decompression.

Table 16   The differential diagnosis of lymphocytic meningitis uncomplicated by significant encephalitis

Condition	Suggestive features
Cerebral tumour	Slow onset Focal neurological signs
Cerebrovascular incidents	Vascular disease elsewhere Signs of pre-existent hypertension Focal neurological signs
Cerebral abscess	Slow onset Possibly focal neurological signs
Degenerative brain disease	Usually a very slow onset (a diagnosis of exclusion)
Meningeal carcinomatosis	
Metabolic diseases	Evidences of diabetes, porphyria etc.
Sarcoidosis	Evidence of sarcoidosis elsewhere Kveim test positive
Subarachnoid haemorrhage	Usually of abrupt onset Subhyaloid haemorrhages
Subdural haematoma	History of head injury Skull fracture Fluctuating mental state

Table 17   Infection related CNS disease associated with a normal or non-specific CSF

Encephalitis lethargica
Malaria
Meningismus
Rabies
Royal Free disease
Worm infections with cerebral involvement
(including cysticercosis and hydatid disease)

INFECTION-RELATED CNS ILLNESSES ASSOCIATED WITH A NORMAL OR
NON-SPECIFIC CSF

Encephalitis lethargica

This is a disease of unknown aetiology and protean manifestations which
commonly occurred in minor epidemics, although sporadic cases occurred.
(Table 17) It is now extremely rare.

Malaria

Any febrile patient who has been in a malarial area should have blood films
examined for malaria. In cerebral malaria (caused by *Plasmodium
falciparum*) parasites are almost invariably present in the peripheral
blood. There may be generalized or focal signs of cerebral dysfunction. The
CSF pressure and protein level are raised and there is a pleocytosis – the
knowledge of the CSF results usually implies a delayed diagnosis!

Meningismus

This is the presence of meningeal signs (Table 13) with a normal CSF in
response to infections usually outside the CNS. Urinary tract infections and
pneumonias are frequent causes – Q fever is often associated with severe
headache and meningeal signs may occur, although the CSF is usually
normal.

Rabies

Rabies is an almost invariably fatal disease usually initiated by the bite of
an infected animal. The incubation period is variable, commonly
1–3 months (range 10–240 days), depending largely upon the dosage and
site of inoculation as the virus travels centripetally via the peripheral nerves
from the site of inoculation to the CNS.

The disease commences with a 2–4 day prodromal period with possible
fever, headache, sore throat, minor mental changes, excessive salivation,
excessive lacrimation or excessive perspiration. Abnormal sensations
present at the inoculation site in about 80% of patients are a major clue to
the diagnosis.

An excitatory phase follows in which anxiety and apprehension become
marked. Muscle tone is generally increased but muscle weakness around
the inoculation site may be present. Cranial nerve palsies and cardiac
dysrhythmias may occur but the classical diagnostic sign is hydrophobia –
a spasmodic contraction of swallowing and respiratory muscles at the taste,
sight, or even sound of water.

A paralytic stage terminates the excitatory phase with progressive generalized flaccid paralysis and preterminal deterioration in conscious level (which is commonly unimpaired until this stage). Occasionally rabies presents with a paralytic illness without an obvious excitation phase.

In a suspected case, the local virus reference laboratory will provide details of the confirmatory tests available. Fluorescent antibody tests and serological tests are available in addition to virus culture from saliva and throat secretions. The differential diagnosis lies between polio and other viral encephalitides, paralysis secondary to an encephalomyelitis caused by rabies vaccination, and hysteria – the latter may occur with an impossibly short incubation period after a bite.

Therapy in an established case is essentially supportive and symptomatic. Several cases of recovery from apparent rabies have been reported and intensive care unit therapy for all sufferers has been advocated.

Pre-exposure prevention by vaccination is possible for those at high risk. Post-exposure prevention, initiated as soon as possible after potential inoculation, rests upon irrigating and washing the bitten area, injection of rabies antiserum intramuscularly and locally, and subsequent vaccination of all exposed patients – including those who have received prophylactic vaccination. The biting animal should be observed if possible: if it does not develop symptoms within 5 days of biting, the chances of it having rabies are minimal. In every case the current WHO recommendations should be consulted.

Reye's syndrome

This is an acute encephalopathy which occurs in association with fatty degeneration of the viscera. The aetiology is unknown but it tends to follow acute viral infections in children including influenza and chickenpox.

The pattern of illness varies considerably. Vomiting is a consistent feature which often begins as the child is recovering from the prodromal illness. Changes in the mental state often progress rapidly to deepening coma, decorticate or decerebrate posturing (Figure 45), flaccidity, fixed dilated pupils and respiratory arrest. Hepatomegaly occurs in about 40% of cases. The CSF commonly shows a normal cell count and protein and liver biopsy provides a definitive diagnosis.

The main differential diagnosis is that of heavy metal poisoning.

Therapy is supportive with treatment of the numerous associated metabolic defects – including hypoglycaemia.

Royal Free Disease (Benign myalgic encephalomyelitis)

This is a disease of disputed aetiology in which relatively minor evidences of neurological dysfunction occur in association with mental symptoms of weakness, lethargy and excess fatigue on exertion. It also seems to elicit a secondary encephalopathy in those who rightly or wrongly dispute its presumed infective aetiology: symptoms include lack of scientific approach to the problem and polemical outbursts.

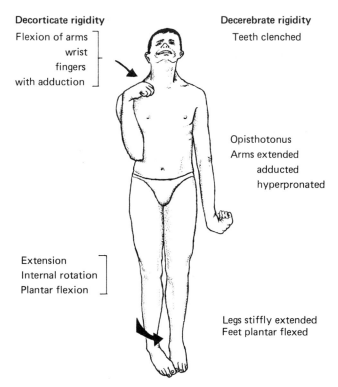

Decorticate rigidity

Flexion of arms ⎤
wrist |
fingers ⊢
with adduction ⎦

Decerebrate rigidity

Teeth clenched

Opisthotonus
Arms extended
adducted
hyperpronated

Extension ⎤
Internal rotation |
Plantar flexion ⎦

Legs stiffly extended
Feet plantar flexed

Figure 45   Typical signs of decorticate and decerebrate rigidity. (Adapted from *Update*, with permission)

SLOW VIRUS INFECTIONS

Slow virus infections are all rare. They usually cause a low grade infection with a long incubation period before symptoms or signs become evident, and thereafter there is usually an inexorable slow deterioration in cerebral function.

Jacob–Creutzfeldt disease

This usually affects older males on a sporadic basis and causes progressive dementia often with multifocal muscle twitching. The causative agent (possibly not a genuine virus) is resistant to several sterilizing procedures and has been transmitted by neurosurgical and ophthalmological instruments.

Kuru

This was a disease localized to a small area of Papua New Guinea inhabited by the Fore people and which presented with a syndrome not unlike multiple sclerosis. It was transmitted by cannibalistic ingestion of the brains of deceased humans.

Progressive multifocal leukoencephalopathy

This may affect immunosuppressed patients with lymphomas, and patients with other chronic disorders. It is a demyelinating disease with progressive neurological abnormalities. It is caused by infection with a papovavirus.

Subacute sclerosing panencephalitis

This is caused by the measles virus and occurs several years after an apparently unremarkable attack of measles. There is progressive neurological deterioration with personality changes, mental deterioration, involuntary movements, seizures and motor abnormalities (Figure 45). Death usually ensues 6–36 months after onset.

COMPLICATIONS OF ACUTE MENINGITIS

In the acute stage *raised intracranial pressure*, coma and death may ensue, particularly in untreated bacterial meningitis. *Epileptic seizures* may occur with their own attendant complications: it seems sensible to treat these with a drug such as phenytoin (which does not interfere with the assessment of the patient's conscious level) after initial treatment with intravenous diazepam. Slow resolution of a meningitis on appropriate therapy, should suggest the formation of *subdural effusions* or *focal collections of pus* as in early abscess formation. *Hydrocephalus* may occur secondary to blockage of CSF pathways and all young children with meningitis should have their skull circumference monitored. *Deafness* may occur and in mumps infection this may be permanent.

Other complications include eye damage, or effects caused by the organism affecting other sites either directly or by immunological mechanisms.

INFECTION-RELATED DISEASES WHICH HAVE THEIR PREDOMINANT EFFECTS ON THE PERIPHERAL NERVOUS SYSTEM (Table 18)

Table 18 Infection related illnesses which have their predominant effects on the peripheral nerves

Botulism	Leprosy
Diphtheria	Polyneuritis
Guillain–Barré syndrome	Tetanus

Infection-related diseases of the nervous system

Botulism

This is a toxin mediated disease in which the toxins inhibit release of acetylcholine at cholinergic synapses, including those of the autonomic preganglionic fibres, parasympathetic postganglionic fibres and those at the neuromuscular junctions. The toxins are produced by *Clostridium botulinum*, an organism which flourishes in anaerobic environments provided by inadequately sterilized or packaged foods. The CNS is unaffected but cranial nerve neuromuscular junctions tend to be involved early and severely.

Illness usually occurs 12–48 hours after ingestion of the toxins (minimum 6 hours): depending on the particular type of toxin involved there may be vomiting or diarrhoea before the onset of neurological symptoms and this may provide a diagnostic clue. However, patients may only present with neurological features and the diagnosis has to be made from these alone. Classically there is acute symmetrical dysfunction of cranial nerves followed by a descending pattern of paralysis involving respiratory, abdominal and limb muscles. Blurred vision, diplopia, dysarthria and dysphagia are common. The conscious level is unimpaired and in common with many toxin mediated illnesses there is no fever in the absence of infective complications. If the patient survives (many do not) recovery is usually complete.

The differential diagnosis includes ingestion of chemical poisons, other toxins or drug reactions: these may have a shorter incubation period. The absence of fever in the uncomplicated acute stage helps exclude poliomyelitis, meningitis and encephalitis. The diagnosis can be confirmed by demonstration of botulinal toxin in the ingested food, in the patient's faeces or serum.

Treatment involves the elimination of residual toxin from the gut by gastric lavage or by purgation. Antitoxin should be administered urgently. Patients with neurological involvement should be urgently admitted to an Intensive Care Unit for monitoring and treatment of respiratory and cardiac dysfunctions. Penicillin has been advocated to eliminate possible organisms from the gut, but this therapy is controversial. Drugs that stimulate acetylcholine release have also been tried.

Diphtheria

In diphtheria neurological manifestations mediated by exotoxin may follow laryngeal, pharyngeal and nasal diphtheria (and occasionally after wound diphtheria in the tropics). The clinical sequence of paralysis reflects the sequential dysfunction of palatal innervation, eye innervation, heart innervation, pharyngeal, laryngeal and respiratory innervation, and finally limb innervation. Paralysis is usually bilateral but one side may be more markedly affected: sensory changes are seldom found.

In pharyngeal paralysis (often in the third week of illness) the patient cannot shut off the mouth from the nose, with resulting difficulty in swallowing and nasal regurgitation of fluids. In ocular paralysis (often in the 3rd–5th week of illness) there is difficulty in accommodation with blurred vision. Occasionally eye muscle paralysis results, especially affecting the external rectus muscle which may result in squint and double vision. In laryngeal paralysis there is loss of voice and an ineffective cough. Paralysis of respiratory muscles, heart muscles and limb muscles require anticipation and early treatment. Recovery if the patient survives is usually complete.

A history of a recent mild sore throat associated with a low grade fever may be crucial in making a correct diagnosis in any patient who presents with any of the above neurological symptoms and signs. Treatment consists of urgent administration of antitoxin in an attempt to prevent further toxin-induced paralysis. Antibacterial therapy (usually penicillin or erythromycin) should be given to eradicate persisting *Corynebacteria*. Palatal paralysis can often be managed with careful feeding. In pharyngeal paralysis oral feeding is contraindicated and use should be made of naso-gastric tube feeding. If pharyngeal paralysis is severe or extends to the larynx, it may be safer to keep the stomach empty and to feed intravenously for a brief period.

Guillain–Barré syndrome (often known as acute infective polyneuritis)

It appears that Schwann cell myelin sheaths in the peripheral nerves are damaged by immunologically activated cells after sensitization associated with a recent infection or recent immunization. Microscopically there is segmental demyelination with oedema, infiltration with mononuclear cells, and in some cases nerve degeneration. Nerve conduction studies show slowing of motor and sensory impulses whilst electromyography shows signs of denervation. In many ways this is similar to post-infectious encephalomyelitis but with emphasis on peripheral nervous system damage.

Symptoms and signs are usually of an acute onset, commonly with a symmetrical flaccid muscular weakness with diminished or absent tendon reflexes, and sensory disturbance which usually involves distal rather than proximal limb segments. This and the pattern of progression plus demonstrable sensory signs may serve to differentiate from poliomyelitis.

In 'infection-related' cases there is an acute febrile prodromal illness followed by distal sensorimotor signs and a paralysis which may affect all four limbs and which classically ascends from the lower limbs. There may be an intermittent progression with a variable, sometimes recurrent course. Respiratory or bulbar paralysis may occur. Papilloedema and other evidence of *central* nervous system involvement occurs in at least 10% of patients.

The CSF classically shows a normal cell count with a disproportionate and marked rise in the protein level, although the classical syndrome has rarely occurred with repeatedly unremarkable CSF changes.

The major differential diagnoses of both acute and chronic polyneuritis are listed in Table 19.

Table 19   **The common aetiologies of polyneuritis**

Aetiology	*Examples*
Collagen/vascular	Systemic lupus erythematosus
Idiopathic	Polyarteritis nodosa, rheumatoid arthritis, sarcoidosis
Deficiency or metabolic	Diabetes, porphyria, pernicious anaemia, amyloidosis, myxoedema
Genetic	Various syndromes
Infection − local complications of generalized infections	Brucellosis, leprosy, syphilis, post-dysenteric, septicaemic, tuberculosis, typhoid, HB$_s$Ag carriers with polyarteritis
Malignant disease	May occur with virtually any neoplasm
Toxic/infective	Post-dysenteric, diphtheria, tetanus
Toxic inorganic substances	Alcohol, heavy metals, drugs
Post-infectious	Guillain-Barré syndrome

Leprosy

This disease has a predilection for the skin and nerves. It may cause both motor and sensory dysfunction and is one of the few conditions that causes nerve thickening. Leprosy should be suspected if there are erythematous or hypopigmented skin lesions with associated hypoanaesthesia and lack of sweating, especially if there is local or non-local nerve thickening or dysfunction. Affected patients almost invariably have spent more than one year in leprosy endemic areas.

Tetanus

Although the pathology affects the spinal cord tissues the manifestations are almost exclusively peripheral and justify the inclusion of tetanus in this section.

Neurological manifestations of tetanus are caused by *Clostridium tetani* exotoxin which suppresses inhibitory influences on motor neurones. The

211

exotoxin also affects neurocirculatory and neuroendocrine pathways. A history of a previous wound may or may not be available and affected patients often have not been immunized against tetanus.

Clinically there may be a brief non-specific prodrome followed by lockjaw or trismus which is characteristic. Intermittent, irregular, unpredictable spasms of bodily muscles may become evident, constituting generalized tetanus which may lead to exhaustion or respiratory embarrassment. Spasm of facial muscles leads to a bizarre almost grinning expression − risus sardonicus. Usually there is persistent muscular hypertonicity, increased tendon reflexes, unimpaired conscious level and low grade fever. There are no sensory signs. In adults tetanus is occasionally limited to particular muscle groups. In neonates tetanus often presents as a failure to suck: this tends to occur in underdeveloped tropical countries and is often secondary to infection of the umbilical stump.

The differential diagnoses include dental abscess (which should be obvious), meningitis, or encephalitis (the CSF in tetanus is usually normal apart from intermittent pressure elevation during muscle spasms). Muscle spasms in rabies may present a problem in differentiation as both may follow animal bites, but rabies characteristically involves muscles of swallowing and trismus is absent. Abdominal rigidity may suggest an intra-abdominal emergency but careful examination should reveal muscle stiffness elsewhere. Hysteria and phenothiazine reactions are also possible differential diagnoses: phenothiazines often cause 'cogwheel' parkinsonian rigidity. Rabies presenting in Britain is always acquired abroad.

Treatment in essence involves urgent administration of antitoxin which, in theory at least, will neutralize circulating toxin (but which will have little effect on toxin already fixed to nervous tissues) and elimination of the source of the toxin if feasible. Antibacterial therapy should also be given. The patient should be nursed in a quiet, darkened room and disturbed as little as possible because the slightest stimulus can precipitate muscle spasms. Intensive supportive care, muscle relaxants, tracheostomy and ventilation may all be required. Autonomic imbalances require expert management.

ABSCESS FORMATION AFFECTING THE NERVOUS SYSTEM

Nervous system abscesses may well enter into the differential diagnosis of infectious diseases because of an association between a febrile illness and neurological features. The sites at which abscess formation can cause neurological dysfunction have been listed in Figure 42. Abscess formation compressing peripheral nerves will cause progressive disability of lower motor neurone characteristics (see Table 12).

Extradural abscesses are usually secondary to skull bone infections and may be difficult to diagnose as focal signs usually only occur if the abscess is large: headache which may be lateralized may be the only symptom of note. Extradural abscess may present as a space occupying lesion which results in spinal cord pressure. There may be signs related to skull bone sepsis.

Intracerebral abscesses are commonly single and evolve through an encephalitic stage to pus formation and then to a stage of walling off. They may be caused by spread of infection from local sources or may be metastatic from a peripheral (perhaps unnoticed) septic focus. Such blood borne infection usually, but by no means always, affects brain supplied by the middle cerebral artery.

Subdural abscesses may follow extradural sepsis after penetration of the dura. The presentation is often with fever, epileptic seizures and focal neurological signs.

Subarachnoid abscess is a rare form of subdural abscess in which pus is limited to the subarachnoid space.

Differentiation between uncomplicated intracerebral abscess from meningitis and encephalitis

A history obtained from the patient or a relative is of paramount importance. A history of head injury is obviously important.

A period of vague ill-defined ill health followed by signs related to a space occupying lesion suggests an abscess (or neoplasm) but occasionally the onset may be sudden or associated with transient symptoms or signs (perhaps related to arrival of embolic infected material). There may also be a source for metastatic dissemination of infection, such as sinusitis, middle ear disease, bronchiectasis, cystic fibrosis with pulmonary sepsis, congenital heart disease or endocarditis. Ear infections classically give rise to abscesses in the temporal lobes or cerebellum; frontal sinusitis is often associated with frontal lobe abscesses.

Lateralized neurological signs are uncommon in *early* meningitis and their presence implies either a focal encephalitis or a space occupying lesion such as an abscess. Rapidly progressive abscesses may be associated with pyrexia and leukocytosis: a slowly progressive abscess may be associated with *neither* fever nor leukocytosis and neoplasm may be initially suspected.

Spinal extradural or epidural abscesses are often caused by blood borne infections or are secondary to vertebral osteomyelitis. Bacteria possibly responsible include staphylococci and *Myco. tuberculosis*. In the early stages there is back pain, fever, leukocytosis and spinal tenderness on gentle percussion. Later, paraplegia or tetraplegia results from either spinal cord compression or interference with spinal cord blood supply. Symptoms depend on the site of the compressing lesion: sensory symptoms usually occur early with root pain, paraesthesiae or temporary hyperaesthesiae made worse by coughing. Motor symptoms usually consist of weakness, stiffness and limb unsteadiness. If the spinal substance of one side is compressed, there will be progressive homolateral lower motor neurone symptoms and signs (Table 12) at the level of compression. Homolateral upper motor neurone signs occur below the level of compression and also on the contralateral side there is loss of pain and temperature sensation. Suspected spinal cord compression is a *neurosurgical emergency.*

All patients with meningitis and an impaired conscious level should have their skull carefully palpated to exclude obvious skull fracture or local tenderness related to sinusitis or mastoiditis.

INVESTIGATIONS IN SUSPECTED NERVOUS SYSTEM INFECTIONS

The indications for and technique of lumbar puncture with the interpretation of CSF findings are detailed in Chapter 15.

In uncomplicated acute onset meningitis the *skull X-ray* should be normal, without asymmetry, unilateral calcifications, evidence of raised intracranial pressure or signs of skull fracture. In subacute or chronic conditions the skull X-ray may show signs of raised intracranial pressure including erosion of the posterior clinoid processes with decalcification of the dorsum sellae, and there may be separation of the cranial sutures in children. If there is a space occupying lesion within the skull the pineal, if calcified, will be seen to be displaced away from the lesion.

An *electroencephalogram* may reveal diffuse abnormality in diffuse lesions such as meningitis but focal lesions such as abscesses or neoplasms may be identified and even characterized.

An *echogram* may reveal evidence of midline displacement or space occupying lesions and isotope brain scans may reveal the size and situation of focal lesions.

Electroneurography or *electromyography* may reveal evidence of nervous or secondary muscle dysfunction secondary to infections affecting the peripheral nervous system.

In certain centres *computerized axial tomography* may be available and can provide identification of quite small abnormalities and in many cases can reliably differentiate between various possible aetiologies: this investigation is replacing the invasive contrast techniques such as carotid angiography or pneumoencephalography.

Suggested further reading

Hoeprich, P.D. (1977). *Infectious Diseases.* (London: Harper and Row)
Walton, J.N. (1977). *Brain's Diseases of the Nervous System.* (Oxford: Oxford University Press)

13
Vomiting and diarrhoea

INTRODUCTION

Understanding of the pathogenesis of vomiting and diarrhoea requires appreciation of gut fluid dynamics (Figure 46). In a healthy state the small bowel is responsible for the secretion and absorption of large volumes of fluid, whereas the large bowel can only make relatively minor absorptive adjustments.

The ileo-caecal valve functions as an anatomical and 'bacteriological' valve: the small bowel normally contains relatively few bacteria compared with the large bowel (Figure 47) and pathogens usually affect predominantly either the small or large bowel.

Occasionally some infections (especially campylobacter, salmonella and yersinia) cause a 'mixed' small and large bowel diarrhoea.

Small bowel diarrhoea

In general *small bowel pathogens* often cause disease by means of toxins and less often by deep invasion of the bowel wall. Such toxins cause secretion of large volumes of water which then pass into the large bowel: if the large bowel is uninflamed it can function as a reservoir and consequently large volumes of rather fluid faeces are passed frequently. Alternatively, as in giardiasis, malabsorption may cause frequent bulky stools.

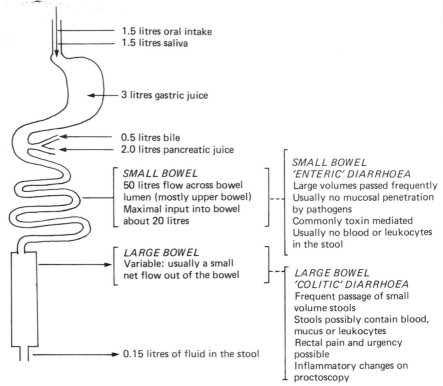

1.5 litres oral intake
1.5 litres saliva

3 litres gastric juice

0.5 litres bile
2.0 litres pancreatic juice

SMALL BOWEL
50 litres flow across bowel
lumen (mostly upper bowel)
Maximal input into bowel
about 20 litres

LARGE BOWEL
Variable: usually a small
net flow out of the bowel

0.15 litres of fluid in the stool

SMALL BOWEL
'ENTERIC' DIARRHOEA
Large volumes passed frequently
Usually no mucosal penetration
by pathogens
Commonly toxin mediated
Usually no blood or leukocytes
in the stool

LARGE BOWEL
'COLITIC' DIARRHOEA
Frequent passage of small
volume stools
Stools possibly contain blood,
mucus or leukocytes
Rectal pain and urgency
possible
Inflammatory changes on
proctoscopy

Figure 46   Adult gastrointestinal fluid dynamics: all figures are approximate daily
amounts

Large bowel diarrhoea

In contrast *large bowel pathogens* often invade the large bowel wall and
thereby cause large bowel irritability. Because of this the bowel cannot
function as an effective reservoir and, as small bowel function is often
relatively preserved, small amounts of less fluid faeces are passed
frequently. Additionally, invasion of the large bowel may cause
inflammatory changes which may result in blood, mucus or pus in the
stool. Rectal pain, 'desperate' urgency or incontinence usually imply large
bowel pathology.

Host defences

Host defences against intestinal infection with pathogenic organisms
include:

Personal hygiene

Simple measures such as handwashing reduce the chances of transfer of
pathogenic organisms to the mouth or to food by contaminated hands.

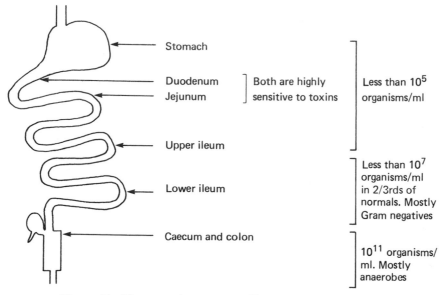

Figure 47   The normal quantities of bacterial flora in the gut

Gastric acidity

Gastric acidity acts as a barrier which ingested intestinal pathogens have to overcome.

Local immunity

This is provided in the bowel by secretory IgA: possibly IgG and IgM may leak into the bowel from inflamed mucosal blood vessels.

Excessive gut motility

This might be considered a defence mechanism, in that vomiting and diarrhoea constitute a socially inconvenient attempt by the gut to rid itself of intestinal pathogens. Interestingly, gastrointestinal pathogens which have a short incubation period often cause predominant vomiting (as if to expel upper gastrointestinal pathogens) whereas those with a longer incubation period often cause predominant diarrhoea (as if the gut realizes that the pathogens have passed so far along the gut that vomiting would not expel the pathogens).

The normal gut flora

This usually prevents overgrowth of potentially pathogenic organisms. Certain antibacterial drugs may disrupt the normal flora allowing catastrophic overgrowth of organisms such as the staphylococci, thereby causing a necrotizing enterocolitis.

217

Breast feeding of infants

This results in a lower incidence of infection-related vomiting and diarrhoea.

Community hygiene

This involves the provision of uncontaminated food and water supplies, safe sewage disposal, and isolation of infected members of the community.

The common infection-related causes of vomiting and diarrhoea are listed in Table 20.

Table 20   The common causes of infection-related vomiting and diarrhoea

Disease in which vomiting is usually an early or predominant feature
    Bacillus cereus food poisoning (short incubation)
    Staphylococcal food poisoning
    Winter vomiting disease

Disease in which diarrhoea is an early or predominant feature
    Amoebic colitis
    Antibacterial drug induced diarrhoea
    Bacillus cereus (long incubation)
    Bacterial overgrowth
    Campylobacter enteritis
    Clostridium perfringens (Type A)
    Enterotoxin-producing *Escherichia coli*
    Giardia lamblia
    Necrotizing enterocolitis
    Pseudomembranous colitis
    Rotavirus
    Shigella
    Tropical sprue
    Vibrio cholerae
    Yersinia enterocolitica

Diseases in which either vomiting or diarrhoea may predominate
    Clostridium botulinum
    Enteroviruses
    Non-typhoidal salmonellae
    Vibrio parahaemolyticus

INFECTIONS IN WHICH VOMITING IS USUALLY A PREDOMINANT FEATURE
(Table 21)

Bacillus cereus food poisoning

This toxin mediated illness classically occurs 1–3 hours after the ingestion of rice in which the organism has been allowed to grow and release its toxin.

Table 21 'Infectious' diseases in which vomiting is usually the predominant feature

Organism	Nature of illness	Usual incubation period	Abdominal pain	Fever	White cell count	Usual duration	Common vehicle of illness
Bacillus cereus (short incubation)	Toxin mediated	Less than 3 hours	Possible	No	Normal	Brief	Rice
Staphylococcal food poisoning	Toxin mediated	1–6 hours	Possible	No	Normal	Less than 24 hours	Food
Winter vomiting disease	Almost certainly viral in most cases	About 2 days Maximum about 7 days	Possible			A few days	

As in most toxin mediated intestinal diseases fever and a raised white cell count are unusual. A predominantly diarrhoeal illness may also occur (see later).

Staphylococcal food poisoning

Abrupt onset vomiting typically occurs within 6 hours of eating a meal in which a toxin-producing *Staphylococcus aureus (pyogenes)* has been allowed to grow. The illness usually lasts less than 24 hours: diarrhoea may occur as a late manifestation but is usually trivial compared with the vomiting. Consistent with the toxin causation there is no fever and in the absence of dehydration the white cell count is usually normal. The major diagnostic clue is the shortness of the incubation period: *Bacillus cereus* food poisoning should be differentiated by the dietary history. Non-typhoidal salmonella infection may have vomiting as an initial feature but usually diarrhoea is predominant.

Both *Bacillus cereus* and staphylococcal food poisoning are caused by ingested toxins and thus affected patients are non-infectious and do not require isolation, although the food responsible will still cause illness.

Winter vomiting disease

This is a syndrome in which certain viruses have been implicated. The syndrome only tends to be recognized when institutional outbreaks occur.

INFECTIONS IN WHICH DIARRHOEA IS USUALLY A PREDOMINANT FEATURE (Table 22)

Amoebic colitis

The causative organism is a protozoa, *Entamoeba histolytica*. Affected patients have usually been to the tropics or subtropics. The incubation

Table 22 Infectious diseases in which diarrhoea is a predominant feature

Organism	Nature of illness	Usual incubation period	Blood in stool	Abdominal pain	Fever	Usual duration	Vehicle/ vector	Other points
Amoebic colitis	Bowel wall invasion	Variable	Usually + mucus	Possible: large bowel type	±	Variable	Cysts in water or food	Usually a history of foreign travel
Campylobacter	Penetration of bowel wall	5–7 days 3–10 possible	In about 40%	Possibly very severe	Usually	Commonly 1–3 days	Animals	
Clostridium perfringens Type A	Toxin mediated	8–16 hours	No	Possible	No	24–28 hours	Cooked meat	Spores resist cooking
Enterotoxin-producing *E. coli*	Enterotoxin	A few days	No	Possible: usually mild	No	Variable: commonly 1–2 days		Causes some infantile and travellers' diarrhoea
Giardia lamblia	Mostly coverage of upper small bowel	Variable: large range	No	Possible: small intestinal	No	Variable	Cysts in water or food	Often tropically derived 'persistent travellers' diarrhoea'
Rotavirus	Infection of bowel wall	1–2 days	Not usually	Possible	±	Less than 1 week		Mostly in the under-fives
Shigella sonnei, flexneri, boydii, dysenteriae	Invasion of large bowel wall	2–4 days 1–7 possible	Very common + mucus	Large bowel type colic	±	A few days Up to 2 weeks rarely	Contacts	*S. dysenteriae* (the cause of classical bacillary dysentery) produces a significant toxin
Vibrio cholerae	Toxin mediated	6–72 hours	No	Colicky	No	1–7 days	Infected water	Organisms have to be present in the small bowel

period of amoebic dysentery ranges from a few days to several months or years: 2–4 weeks is common. It may have an abrupt onset or it may start insidiously, become chronic, and be confused with 'idiopathic' ulcerative colitis. Amoebic dysentery is an invasive colitic illness with bloody diarrhoea. On proctoscopy amoebic ulcers may be seen: they usually have undermined edges and the intervening bowel wall is normal in appearance. Microscopy of the stool or rectal mucus may reveal actively mobile amoebae. Treatment is with metronidazole which usually kills the invading amoebae, but a subsequent course of diloxanide furoate is necessary to eliminate persisting interluminal amoebae.

Antibacterial drug induced diarrhoea

Diarrhoea is a not uncommon complication of antibacterial therapy and, necrotizing enterocolitis and pseudomembranous colitis apart, is usually a trivial illness caused by a postulated disturbance of the normal flora or by a specific effect of the antibacterial drug on the gut. The antibacterial drug implicated should be discontinued *and* consideration given to the possibility that the disease for which it was given might have been the cause of the diarrhoea.

Bacillus cereus

In its longer incubation period illness (usually about 10 hours) there may be diarrhoea with tenesmus. Fever and vomiting are uncommon and the illness usually lasts about 12 hours.

Bacterial proliferation in an anatomically abnormal small bowel

This may occur in blind loops, diverticulae or proximal to obstructing lesions.

Campylobacter

This infection often seems to be acquired from animals or animal products. The average incubation period is 3–5 days. Fever and prodromal rigors may occur, presumably in relation to transitory bacteraemia. Abdominal pain, which may be severe enough to suggest a surgical emergency, is a very suggestive feature.

Clostridium perfringens (welchi) (Type A)

This organism produces an enterotoxin mediated illness with an incubation period of 8–16 hours from the time of ingestion of the food in which the organism has released its toxin. If vomiting (which is unusual) occurs the longer incubation period distinguishes from staphylococcal or *Bacillus cereus* food poisoning. Classically there is little or no fever, a normal white cell count and no blood in the stool. The illness usually lasts 24–28 hours.

Enterotoxin-producing Escherichia coli

These illnesses present with a fairly abrupt onset of watery diarrhoea. The incubation period appears to be a few days and the duration, although variable, is often 1–2 days, but certain serotypes may produce a very protracted illness. *E. coli* produces a mild illness at present but in the past outbreaks were associated with a disturbing mortality rate.

Toxin production is not confined to the classical 'enteropathogenic' serotypes as the ability to produce certain toxins can be transmitted by plasmids to other *E. coli* serotypes.

Toxin-producing *E. coli* are often implicated in infantile diarrhoea and the common transient travellers' diarrhoea.

Although toxin mediated a minor degree of bowel wall invasion may occur as there may be an initial low grade fever.

Invasive Escherichia coli

Certain serotypes of *E. coli* may produce a shigella-like illness with diarrhoea, abdominal pain, tenesmus and a 'large bowel type' stool. As might be predicted from the invasive nature of the infection fever is often present.

Giardia lamblia

This protozoan organism causes diarrhoea by its presence on the surface of the upper small bowel and by associated changes which affect the absorptive villi. In symptomatic cases there is a malabsorption-like syndrome which, in addition to the diarrhoea, often produces upper gastrointestinal symptoms including anorexia and nausea: a feeling of bloating after food is particularly suggestive of giardiasis. Giardia is the most common cause of *persistent* travellers' diarrhoea.

The diagnosis is usually made by finding giardia cysts on stool microscopy: on occasion aspiration of upper small bowel fluid is necessary to visualize the motile protozoa themselves. Metronidazole is effective and (apart from alcohol intolerance) is remarkably free from side-effects in the dosages used against giardia.

Necrotizing enterocolitis

This severe disease classically affects very young infants who may, or may not, have received prior antibacterial therapy: there is a sudden onset of colitic diarrhoea and vomiting. Staphylococcal overgrowth in the bowel is often implicated but a similar syndrome may occur with overgrowth of other bacteria.

Pseudomembranous colitis

There is a spectrum of disease severity. In severe forms this disease may be responsible for much morbidity and mortality, whereas mild illnesses may not be recognized or merely dismissed as 'trivial antibacterial drug associated diarrhoea'. In its severe (and therefore recognized) forms this illness may affect any age group and is often associated with prior anti-bacterial therapy or surgical operations.

The symptoms and signs are caused by the liberation of a toxin from *Clostridium difficile*. The pseudomembrane produced in the large bowel is visualized sigmoidoscopically as a raised film or plaque of greyish/whitish/yellowish colour. Treatment consists of withdrawal of any antibacterial therapy which might have precipitated the illness, in association with vigorous supportive therapy. Antibacterial agents such as oral vancomycin have been used successfully and steroids may have to be used.

Rotavirus

This organism is a major cause of non-bacterial diarrhoea, particularly affecting children under 5 years of age during the winter months. The incubation period is commonly 1–2 days and the illness usually lasts less than one week. Diarrhoea results from impaired function of the upper small bowel absorptive mechanisms.

A low grade fever may be present but there is no blood in the stool and the white cell count is usually normal. Associated respiratory tract symptoms are present in about half the children affected. In the initial stages vomiting is common but overall diarrhoea is predominant.

Shigella (bacillary) dysentery

These organisms produce a large bowel type diarrhoea with frequent small volume stools which may contain blood, mucus or pus. In the very early stages the diarrhoea may be profuse and watery. Fever, abdominal cramps and tenesmus may be present and 'idiopathic' ulcerative colitis may be simulated. In contrast with amoebic dysentery shigella colitis tends to have a more abrupt onset and stool microscopy reveals many polymorpho-nuclear leukocytes (in amoebic dysentery such leukocytes are not common).

Spread is faecal–oral and the infecting dose of the organism is low, largely due to the relative resistance of these organisms to gastric acid. The incubation period is usually 2–4 days (1–7 possible). The illnesses produced are usually self-limiting, generally lasting 2–7 days, although the more severe forms may last about 2 weeks or more. Illness may be very severe, especially if due to S. *dysenteriae* which, in addition to bowel wall invasion, produces a pathologically relevant enterotoxin.

In Britain S. *sonnei* and S. *flexneri* are the commonest species isolated: S. *flexneri*, S. *boydii* and S. *dysenteriae* are mostly imported infections. Despite the lack of extracolonic invasion meningism and (allergic) post-dysenteric arthritis may occur, especially if the patient has histocompatibility antigen HLA B 27.

In general it is best to withhold antibacterial therapy in mild illness but if illness is severe most physicians would prescribe an appropriate antibacterial drug. If the patient is fit enough to remain outside hospital antibacterial therapy is probably not indicated.

Tropical sprue

This disease affects patients who have been abroad, usually to the tropics or subtropics: interestingly there are particular areas where sprue is common. There is chronic malabsorption with steatorrhoea leading to weight loss with various deficiencies, particularly of iron and folate. The exact pathogenesis is uncertain but large bowel bacteria (particularly *E. coli* and *bacteroides*) colonize the small bowel. Damage to small bowel villi results and malabsorption ensues. Foods which should be absorbed are not, and therefore pass into the large bowel leading to further bacterial proliferation which promotes retrograde colonization of the small bowel and a vicious circle is achieved. In addition bile salts are deconjugated by the colonizing bacteria and the resulting bile compounds irritate the large bowel to cause ('choluretic') diarrhoea.

Diagnosis is by demonstration of malabsorption and by small bowel biopsy which shows characteristic appearances which serve to differentiate sprue from coeliac disease. Simultaneous aspiration of upper small bowel fluid will allow giardiasis to be excluded. Treatment is with antibacterial drugs, commonly tetracyclines, and correction of the relevant deficiencies.

Vibrio cholera

The cholera vibrio is usually transmitted by water which has been contaminated with infected faeces. After an incubation period of 6–72 hours there is a profuse enterotoxin-mediated small bowel diarrhoea which lasts for 1–7 days unless death supervenes. In classical cholera large volumes of isotonic rice water stools are passed, leading to severe dehydration. In the absence of complications such as severe dehydration there is no fever, no elevation of the white cell count and no blood in the stool.

Vibrios have to be present in the small bowel in order to initiate the cholera syndrome and antibacterial therapy, usually with a tetracycline, may be used in conjunction with rapid and adequate fluid replacement.

Yersinia enterocolitica

In Britain this is an uncommon pathogen. It may cause a diarrhoeal illness in which abdominal pain, leukocytosis and vomiting (as a relatively minor feature) may occur. It is basically an invasive illness with intestinal ulceration particularly in the terminal ileum. Given this combination of symptoms and signs it is not surprising that it may simulate appendicitis.

Travellers' diarrhoea

Diarrhoea is an extremely common occurrence in travellers to foreign lands. Fortunately most attacks are of short duration and aggressive treatment is therefore not indicated. It is likely that most episodes are caused by the acquisition of indigenous toxin-producing strains of *E. coli* which interestingly are often *not* classical enteropathogenic serotypes. Presumably the local inhabitants, and the traveller after recovery, are immune to the particular toxin responsible. Prevention of travellers' diarrhoea involves the use of 'domestic precautions' as detailed in Chapter 14. In addition pretravel vaccination against cholera or typhoid might be considered, and in areas of particular risk tetracyclines can be used prophylactically against cholera. Of many preparations that have been advocated for travellers' diarrhoea Streptotriad, a combination of streptomycin and three sulphonamides, appears to be the most useful drug for countering organisms that are sensitive to these drugs (many organisms are not). It would seem sensible to reserve it for short term usage only.

INFECTIONS IN WHICH EITHER VOMITING OR DIARRHOEA MAY PREDOMINATE (Table 23)

In infants almost any non-enteric infection may present with vomiting or diarrhoea as a possible symptom. Prominent among those that may do so are otitis media, meningitis and pyelonephritis.

Clostridium botulinum

After a brief illness (in which vomiting or diarrhoea may or may not occur) neurological manifestations develop. Typically a symmetrical descending paralysis without sensory symptoms or signs commences about 12−48 hours after eating inadequately tinned or bottled foods in which the organism has grown and formed the toxin. It is a very rare disease.

Enteroviruses

Polio, Echo and coxsackie viruses may each cause relatively minor gastrointestinal upsets with or without further manifestations.

Table 23 Infectious diseases in which either vomiting or diarrhoea may predominate

	Non-typhoidal salmonellae*		Typhoid fever †	Vibrio parahaemolyticus
	Food poisoning	Bloodstream invasion		
Nature of illness	Toxins + irritation	Septicaemia + or − focal lesions	Septicaemic + focal lesions	Damage to bowel wall
Usual incubation period	12–48 hours (6–72 possible)	Variable	10–16 days: larger range possible	8–24 hours
Blood in stool	About 30%	Variable	In week 2–3 of illness	Possible
Abdominal pain	Colicky	Variable	Usually vague: watch for perforation	Colicky
Fever	Usually low-grade	Usually high-grade	Present	Common
Usual duration	About 3–4 days	Variable	3–4 weeks: variable	1–2 days
Vehicle/vector	Food or contacts	Food or contacts	Human bodily products	Seafood
Other points	Very common	Focal symptoms and signs may be absent	Commonly acquired abroad: a human excretor of the organism is always responsible	

*Paratyphoid infection may exhibit features of either or both
†Typhoid fever is not a cause of abrupt onset vomiting and diarrhoea in previously well patients

Vomiting and diarrhoea

Malaria

If a patient has been in a malarial area and has a febrile illness blood films *must* be examined to exclude malaria. Gastrointestinal symptoms are a not uncommon manifestation of malaria.

Salmonella infections

These organisms produce three main clinical syndromes:

(1) *Gastro-entero-colitic syndromes.* ('Salmonella food poisoning.: 'Salmonella gastroenteritis').

These syndromes may be produced by one of the 1800 or so named salmonella organisms. The pathogenic mechanisms are variable and depend on the particular organism involved: some organisms produce illness predominantly by invasion of the gut, other organisms may produce toxins and other organisms by a combination of both mechanisms. The incubation period is variable depending on the infecting dose and the particular organism involved, but an incubation period of 12–48 hours is typical. The duration of such syndromes is similarly variable: in the absence of complications the duration is usually 3–4 days, but gastrointestinal S. *paratyphi* infection affecting the gut may cause more protracted diarrhoea. Infection is often derived from food containing the organism: patients with diarrhoea excrete large numbers of organisms in an uncontrolled fashion and may cause marked environmental contamination. Fever, if present, tends to be low grade. The white cell count (if the organism is confined to the gut) is usually normal or only slightly raised.

Occasionally there may be a brief bout of vomiting or diarrhoea at the circumstantial time of acquisition of S. *typhi*: apart from this typhoid is primarily a septicaemic illness, although diarrhoea may be a late feature (with 'peasoup' faeces) if ileal involvement is severe.

(2) *Septicaemic syndromes.* Septicaemic salmonellosis may occur with or without focal intestinal manifestations. Although any of the named salmonella organisms may enter the blood, certain of them tend to persist and, if the patient is unwell with a septicaemic illness, antibacterial therapy should be prescribed, although the effect is often not dramatic.

(3) *Enteric fever syndromes.* These are caused by S. *typhi*, S. *paratyphoid A, B or C.* They are described in Chapter 2.

Vibrio parahaemolyticus

This is commonly a seafood-borne organism and is a common

cause of vomiting and diarrhoea in Japan but it is an uncommon infection in Britain. The incubation period is usually 8–24 hours and the duration of symptoms is variable, usually 1–2 days. It is thought that this illness, in contrast to cholera, is caused predominantly by damage to the gut mucosa rather than by toxin mediated mechanisms.

Infection of the gut with worms

Worm infections of the gut occasionally cause symptoms related to the gastrointestinal tract. Ascaris worms may cause intestinal or biliary tract obstruction, *Strongyloides* infection may cause a duodenitis and diarrhoea, whereas tapeworms are usually asymptomatic – the patient occasionally noting the passage of segments in his stool. In Britain the most common symptom is that of horror when told of the (usually asymptomatic) infection.

Other infections

Viral illnesses, particularly hepatitis, may cause transitory gastrointestinal symptoms in their prodromal periods. Measles may also do so in the malnourished. 'Gastric flu' rarely, if ever, occurs.

THE DIFFERENTIAL DIAGNOSIS OF INFECTION-RELATED VOMITING AND DIARRHOEA

The coincidence of abrupt onset vomiting and diarrhoea is highly suggestive of an infective causation, and if contacts are similarly afflicted the circumstantial evidence is strengthened.

Vomiting alone has many causes: abrupt onset of profuse vomiting in previously well patients suggests staphylococcal or *Bacillus cereus* food poisoning. Non-infectious causes of abrupt onset vomiting include exacerbations of peptic ulcers, gastritis or reactions to substances other than bacterial toxins.

Infantile pyloric stenosis may present with a vomiting illness. It is most frequent in first-born male infants and commonly presents with forceful projectile vomiting in the 4th–6th week of life. Visible peristaltic waves may be seen passing across the epigastrium from left to right. The diagnosis is confirmed by feeling a 1–3 cm diameter lump in the epigastrium which is especially prominent after feeding.

Pregnancy should not be forgotten as a cause of vomiting.

Chronic recurrent vomiting is unlikely to be due to infection.

Diarrhoea alone is more of a diagnostic problem. With the possible exceptions of amoebic colitis, giardiasis and tropical sprue, most infective diarrhoeas tend to be of a rapid onset, rarely persist for longer than about 4 weeks, and are unlikely to produce a diarrhoeal illness of progressive severity over such a period.

NON-INFECTIOUS DIARRHOEAS WHICH MAY SIMULATE INFECTION-RELATED DIARRHOEA

The following non-infective illnesses may simulate infection-related diarrhoea:

Carcinoma of the large bowel

This rarely presents with a brief history of rapid onset diarrhoea.

Diverticulitis

This usually occurs when there is stasis within a large bowel diverticulum, leading to 'focal overgrowth' of large bowel organisms causing bowel wall irritation and diarrhoea. Diarrhoea and fever may occur, lower abdominal pain is common and signs of peritoneal irritation may be present. Rectal bleeding may occur.

Faulty infant feeding

This is perhaps a more common cause of gastrointestinal symptoms in infants than is generally appreciated.

Hirschsprung's disease

This may occasionally present with a severe 'enterocolitic' illness secondary to abnormal bacterial activity proximal to the aganglionic bowel segment.

Hypotension

Hypotension may cause vomiting and diarrhoea. Myocardial infarction, pulmonary embolism or Addison's disease should spring to mind as possible causes for hypotension.

Idiosyncratic responses to foodstuffs

This may cause vomiting or diarrhoea: curry seems to be a frequent offender (personal observation).

Intussusception

One portion of the gut is invaginated into the next portion: it particularly occurs in babies between the ages of 3 and 12 months. There are bouts of abrupt onset severe abdominal pain such that the legs are drawn up and the child becomes pale. Vomiting may be an early symptom and the stools may be loose: blood in the stool ('redcurrant jelly') may be a feature but this is a late sign unless the intussusception is in the distal bowel.

Ischaemic colitis

This usually presents with abrupt onset abdominal pain (usually left sided) and darkish red clots or mucus in the stool. Fever and leukocytosis are usually evident. The presence of vascular disease elsewhere is supportive but not diagnostic evidence.

Laxative abuse

This should be excluded by tactful but direct questioning.

Melaena

Bleeding from an upper gastrointestinal source may present with diarrhoea (as intraluminal blood tends to cause intestinal hurry) but a competent history and examination should exclude this possibility.

Osmotic diarrhoea

This may occur in infants fed with hypertonic feeding solutions which draw fluid into the bowel thereby causing diarrhoea. It may also occur in debilitated adults fed by naso-gastric tube. In both these patient groups the compensatory mechanisms of thirst cannot be exhibited.

Spurious diarrhoea

Faecal impaction may cause an 'overflow' diarrhoea. It is most common in the elderly.

Ulcerative colitis or Crohn's disease

These can present with an abrupt onset diarrhoeal illness. The diagnosis of these 'idiopathic' disorders may be made clinically if there are coincidental 'peripheral' stigmata such as iritis, uveitis, erythema nodosum, sacroilitis or perianal Crohn's lesions. Occasionally gastrointestinal infections appear to trigger off ulcerative colitis or Crohn's disease.

A rectal examination should be performed on all patients in whom an infective aetiology seems unlikely.

Identification of causative organisms

Confirmation of the clinical diagnosis in vomiting or diarrhoea caused by bacterial pathogens depends upon culture of the vomit, stool or implicated food (if available), or identification of toxins in the stool. Protozoal or other parasitic infections are diagnosed by stool examination for the parasites themselves, their ova or their cysts. In the laboratory, growth on special media differentiates those organisms which are likely to cause vomiting and diarrhoea from the normal stool flora. Put more expressively, the large bowel of even the prettiest girl can be likened to a sewer in that it contains a large number of organisms which would be irrelevant to gastrointestinal symptoms, and thus a bacteriologist has to search *selectively* for likely pathogens. The fact that no pathogens are isolated does not necessarily mean that an infectious agent has been excluded, or that the patient is non-infectious.

THEORETICAL BACKGROUND TO FLUID AND ELECTROLYTE BALANCE

Vomiting or diarrhoea leads to water depletion and electrolyte disturbances. There are *two* major causes of water depletion – water depletion *or* sodium depletion, although in practice the two causes often co-exist.

The clinical and biochemical manifestations depend on the pattern of water and electrolyte loss and the ensuing osmotic interrelationships established between the intracellular fluid (ICF) and the extracellular fluid (ECF). The latter comprises the blood plasma and interstitial fluids. Other relevant factors in the management of fluid balance include the acid–base balance, the potassium balance, energy requirements, the renal responses to the various imbalances and the route by which therapy is given.

Osmolarity is the tendency for water to move through a semi-permeable barrier *from* a weaker *to* a stronger solution: the osmolarity of a solution reflects the concentration of solute particles dissolved in a solvent. In human fluid balance the relevant solutes are predominantly electrolytes and proteins, and the solvent is water.

In short term vomiting or diarrhoea the quantity of ICF and ECF protein usually remains static and thus major changes in ICF or ECF osmolarity occur when there are quantitative changes in electrolytes or water content of a solution. Sodium is the major electrolyte concerned in osmotic regulation and, as both sodium and water can travel rapidly between the ECF and the ICF, it is apparent that sodium and water balance are the major determinants of osmotic interrelationships.

231

In pure water depletion the ECF becomes hypertonic and, in an attempt to restore osmotic balance, *water is drawn from the cells* to dilute the ECF. The cells thus become hypertonic – a state of predominant *intracellular* water depletion – which is associated with thirst. The cells also attempt to relieve their hypertonicity by pushing out potassium into the ECF.

In pure sodium depletion the osmotic pressure of the ECF falls and *water is drawn into the cells* from the ECF. The cells are not water depleted and thirst is therefore not a feature. The water depletion is therefore predominantly *extracellular*.

If *combined* sodium and water loss is treated with water alone the ECF osmotic pressure will fall, hyponatraemia will result, and the cells will become bloated because they will have taken up water osmotically from the ECF.

Acid–base balance

Acidosis usually occurs in predominant diarrhoea because diarrhoea is usually alkaline and a metabolic acidosis remains. In severe acidosis symptoms include increased depth and frequency of respiration, mental slowness, vomiting and (somewhat paradoxically in the circumstances) a diuresis. Further water depletion results from increased respiratory loss of water, vomiting, diuresis and decreased oral intake of water.

Alkalosis would be expected if there were predominant vomiting because vomit is usually acidic, and vomiting alone would therefore 'leave' a residual metabolic alkalosis. However, persisting and predominant vomiting is unusual in vomiting of infective aetiology.

Potassium balance

Both vomit and diarrhoea usually have a higher potassium content than that of plasma. Each therefore causes a net potassium deficit and might cause a fall in serum potassium. However, the illness-induced stress response of increased endogenous catabolism will release extra potassium into the ECF and this may counterbalance the loss from the serum: the serum potassium may thus remain deceptively normal despite a net bodily deficit.

Energy balance

Glucose is required for effective absorption of both sodium and water from the upper small bowel. However a major danger for patients with water depletion is the administration of hyperosmolar sugary solutions which perpetuate diarrhoea by drawing even more water into the bowel. In infants carbohydrate malabsorption may occur in any diarrhoeal illness and if large volumes of milk are given the carbohydrate content will not be absorbed but will remain in the gut: water will then be drawn into the bowel by osmotic means, thus perpetuating diarrhoea.

Renal balance in vomiting and diarrhoea

Both water and sodium loss may lead to nitrogen retention and cause a rise in the blood urea level. In any water depleted patient with a raised blood urea level, it is important to discover whether the kidneys are functioning normally and, if they are not functioning normally, whether the renal impairment is intrinsic or extrinsic. Any intrinsic renal disease, particularly acute renal failure, will affect the volume of water that can safely be given and its electrolyte content.

To differentiate between extrinsic and intrinsic renal failure the following principles are of relevance:

(1) In the *absence* of intrinsic renal disease and in the presence of water depletion the kidneys excrete urea in normal or supranormal amounts.

(2) If there *is* intrinsic renal disease the kidneys may not be able to effectively excrete urea.

(3) Normal kidneys in the presence of water depletion causing a raised blood urea will excrete more than 330 mmol/l of urea in the urine if the blood urea is 17 mmol/l or more (unless there is an alkalosis). Put another way, water depleted but otherwise normal kidneys will be able to excrete urea such that the urine urea : plasma urea ratio will exceed 10 : 1.

(4) Intrinsically diseased kidneys will be unable to excrete this much urea and the ratio will be less than 10 : 1. (The same ratios apply if plasma and urinary creatinine are compared.) At a greater level of investigatory capability, the urine : plasma osmolarity ratio in uncomplicated water depletion will be greater than 1.5 : 1, but in the presence of intrinsic renal disease the urine : plasma ratio will be less than 1 : 1.1.

Compared with adults, infants require a proportionally greater daily water intake because:

(1) The infant kidney is exposed to greater stress than the adult kidney – infant kidneys are less efficient homeostatic mechanisms which cannot select and preserve electrolytes as well as adult kidneys.

(2) Infants have a higher respiratory rate with a proportionally larger pulmonary water loss.

(3) The infant surface area : body weight ratio is higher causing a proportionally greater perspiration related fluid loss.

(4) Infants have a higher metabolic rate.

Routes of therapy

In the vast majority of patients cessation of all food or milk intake plus prompt administration of water-based oral replacement clear fluids results in cessation of vomiting. Vomiting of non-toxin origin is often perpetuated by acidosis and volume depletion: therapy with clear fluids will thus disrupt the self-perpetuating cycle of volume depletion-acidosis-vomiting-volume depletion.

CLINICAL ASSESSMENT OF WATER AND METABOLITE BALANCE

Assessment of water depletion

The duration and reported severity of the patient's symptoms provides only an approximate guide to water and electrolyte losses as it is often unclear exactly how much food or water the patient was able to retain.

The degree of water depletion can often be estimated from the computed or previously known body weight: in a recent onset vomiting or diarrhoea a known fall in body weight usually reflects water loss and for practical purposes 1 kg weight loss reflects 1 litre water loss.

Less than 5% water loss causes thirst, dry mucous membranes and loss of skin elasticity.

Five to ten per cent water loss produces severe thirst, marked loss of skin elasticity, oliguria and, in severe cases, stupor and coma.

Water loss of 10% or more produces inadequacy of the circulation (shock) with attendant complications, morbidity and mortality.

Other signs of water depletion in infants include irritability, restlessness, sunken eyes, clouded corneal appearances and a sunken fontanelle in those under about 12 months of age.

A bulging fontanelle with signs of water depletion elsewhere should suggest meningitis.

Assessment of metabolite imbalance

The presence of electrolyte imbalance may be suggested by various clinical tests, side room urinalysis and measurement of urinary specific gravity:

(1) An increased depth and rate of respiration suggests acidosis.
(2) Skeletal muscle weakness and diminished tendon reflexes suggests hypokalaemia, as does abdominal distension and diminished bowel sounds. An electrocardiogram may reveal changes of potassium depletion.
(3) Cerebral dysfunction in infants (including confusion, mental dullness, apathy, coma or fits) suggests hypernatraemia as does the presence of conjunctival suffusion.
(4) Bilirubinuria or excessive urobilinogenuria may suggest that the gastrointestinal upset is part of a hepatitis prodrome.

(5) Proteinuria, haematuria, tubular casts or brown pigmented granular casts may suggest that acute renal failure has complicated the water depletion. Microscopy of the urine may also reveal white cells and organisms suggesting urinary tract infection.

(6) Glycosuria may suggest previously unsuspected hyperglycaemia.

(7) Ketonuria may reflect starvation or diabetic ketosis.

THE PRACTICAL APPROACH TO THERAPY IN PATIENTS WITH VOMITING AND DIARRHOEA OF INFECTIVE AETIOLOGY

Except where previously indicated antibacterial therapy has little to offer in the therapy of infection-related vomiting and diarrhoea: replacement and supportive therapy is therefore the order of the day. As far as symptomatic therapy is concerned bed-rest often relieves colic and anti-peristaltic drugs may be used if symptoms are severe: these drugs do *not* replace the need for fluid therapy and indeed their use may delay the evacuation of pathogenic organisms from the gut or predispose to 'toxic' dilatation of the gut. Antiperistaltic drugs which are commonly used include codeine phosphate, mist. kaolin et morphe, diphenoxylate (Lomotil) and loperamide (Imodium).

In *brief duration* vomiting or diarrhoea in a *previously well* person frequent electrolyte determinations and elaborate calculations are rarely necessary for assessment, diagnosis or treatment. There is *no need* to needle previously well afebrile young children with mild diarrhoea who are admitted to hospital primarily for social reasons *unless* coincidental pathology is suspected.

Hospital management

Knowledge of the normal water balance values is essential before relevant losses and replacement fluids can be computed: Table 24 details the average daily water turnover of normal 70 kg adults and Table 25 the daily 'basal' water requirements of normal subjects in ml/kg at various ages.

Table 24 **Average daily water turnover of a normal adult weighing 70 kg**
Adapted from Wolf, A. V. (1958). *Thirst*. (Springfield: Charles C. Thomas)

| | *Water intake* (ml) | | | *Water output* (ml) | |
	Obligatory	*Facultative*		*Obligatory*	*Facultative*
Drink	650 }	1000	Urine	700 }	1000
Food	750 }		Skin	500 }	
Metabolic	350		Lungs	400	
			Faeces	150	
Subtotal	1750	1000	Subtotal	1750	1000
TOTAL		2750	TOTAL		2750

Table 25   The daily water requirements at various ages under normal conditions.

Age	Body weight (kg)	Estimated water requirements (ml/kg)
3 days	3.0	80–100
10 days	3.2	125–150
3 months	5.4	140–160
6 months	7.3	130–155
9 months	8.6	125–145
1 year	9.5	120–135
2 years	11.8	115–125
4 years	16.2	100–110
6 years	20.0	90–100
10 years	28.7	70–85
14 years	45	50–60
18 years	54	40–50
Adults	70	21–43

As insensible loss varies with the surface area the daily water requirements can also be estimated if the surface area is known: average requirements are 1500 ml/m^2, the minimum requirement being 870 ml/m^2

Table 26   Anticipated 24 hour water requirement in 70 kg adults with vomiting or diarrhoea

Basal requirement for normals (BRN) (See Table 25)   *plus*

Vomit volume (Hopefully nil)   *plus*

Diarrhoea volume (Usually uncertain)   *plus*

Pulmonary loss*   *plus*

Fever loss†   *plus*

Perspiration loss‡   *plus*

TOTAL

*Add 10% of BRN if there is obvious but mild hyperventilation
†Add 20% of BRN for each °C sustained rise in temperature
‡Add 10% of BRN if there is mild perspiration, 20% if there is moderate perspiration, or 1000 ml if there is whole body perspiration. (Obviously the environmental temperature and humidity may affect these figures.)

The major short term considerations in fluid balance are water loss replacement, electrolyte loss replacement, acid–base balance, calorie administration and the route by which these should be administered.

Water loss replacement

(1)   *Estimate the existing water deficit* using signs of dehydration and known or computed weight loss as detailed previously. Aim to replace this loss within 12 hours or less: rates of 500–1000 ml per hour may be used initially if patients have signs of water depletion.

Providing *early* fluid replacement is started promptly, complications such as renal impairment can be averted.

(2) *Estimate the next 24 hours water requirements* (basal requirements plus other anticipated losses) and aim to administer this volume of water within the next 24 hours – see Table 26.

Volume 1 plus volume 2 should be given over the next 24 hours. The calculations can be repeated every 24 hours but in rapidly changing situations overall balance should be reviewed every few hours. Accurate charting of continuing water losses on a fluid balance chart is essential (Table 27).

Blood, plasma or a plasma substitute should be used to restore the blood volume rapidly if patients are hypotensive: for infants an appropriate rate of administration would be 22 ml/kg over 2–4 hours.

Table 27   Relevant parameters in the assessment of continuing fluid losses

	Total intake (Oral, intravenous, intragastric, sub- cutaneous etc.)	*Total output* Known (urine, vomit, diarrhoea) plus Estimated insensible losses (pulmonary, fever and perspiration).	*Running balance*	*Weight in kg*
DAY 1*				
DAY 2*				
DAY 3*				
Etc.				

*In a dynamic situation these times can be shortened to 6 hourly.

Electrolyte loss replacement

Total electrolyte losses may be difficult to quantify in contrast to the readily assayed levels in the serum.

Sodium balance: in *hyponatraemia* the kidneys should be able to excrete excessive water providing adequate fluid supplements are given as isotonic or slightly less than isotonic sodium solutions. *Normonatraemia* can be treated with similar solutions for the same reasons. *Hypernatraemia* has to be treated with a slightly less than isotonic sodium solution given *slowly*: too rapid correction of hypernatraemia by very hypotonic solutions would cause cerebral oedema as water would be drawn osmotically from the diluted blood into the brain (which would still have a high sodium content).

Potassium balance – potassium depletion requires supplementation. For reasons outlined previously the serum potassium may be normal despite a net bodily deficit. In *brief duration* illnesses in *previously well* infants and young adults the serum potassium is rarely of crucial importance – these patients are rarely vulnerable to mild hypokalaemia because they have patient coronary arteries and have not been taking diuretics or digoxin: for them a replacement fluid containing a small amount of potassium is therefore ideal. When dealing with older patients, especially those taking digoxin or diuretics, the serum potassium must be kept strictly within normal limits. Both normokalaemia and mild potassium depletion can be treated initially with a solution containing a small amount of potassium.

Acid–base balance – Any subclinical acidosis will be corrected by the kidneys if intrinsic renal function is unimpaired and if water, sodium and potassium replacement is adequate. For initial oral therapy a solution containing a small amount of bicarbonate would be appropriate.

In adults with severe electrolyte or acid–base imbalance requiring rapid reversal the total quantity of a replacement electrolyte required in mmol/l can be estimated by using the formula:

$$\text{Body weight in kg} \times \left(\begin{array}{c}\text{the ideal } - \text{ actual serum}\\ \text{concentration in mmol/l}\end{array}\right) \times \frac{15}{100}$$

This formula makes use of the fact that the ECF is approximately 15% of the body weight.

Except in exceptional circumstances no more than 15 mmol of potassium should be given in any one hour. After the appropriate electrolyte replacement quantity has been infused the serum electrolytes should be measured and further correction made if necessary.*

Calorie administration

In all but the most transient episodes of vomiting and diarrhoea the provision of energy becomes essential. It is difficult to supply large amounts of energy by mouth without having to give hyperosmolar solutions – which are contraindicated. Remember that isotonic dextrose solution only contains 200 cal/l of energy.

Route of fluid replacement

Fluid replacement by mouth is nearly always successful if given early in the course of illness. Give small amounts of fluid often, rather than large amounts infrequently. If for any reason oral replacement is not possible or absorption of fluid is dubious a brief period of intravenous therapy would be advisable before reintroducing oral therapy. On occasion intragastric fluids by naso-gastric tube may be indicated.

*As an aid to calculation of relevant volumes the normal (i.e. isotonic 'physiological' saline contains 154 mmol/l of sodium and 8.4% sodium bicarbonate contains 1000 mmol/l of bicarbonate.

Table 28 Some possible solutions for management of vomiting and diarrhoea

Solutions	Electrolytes in mmol/l				Energy in cal/l	Osmolarity in mmol/l
	Sodium	Potassium	Chloride	Bicarbonate		
The 'ideal' oral solution* (320 mmol/l)	90	20	80	30	110	320
Half strength oral Hartmann's solution	65.5	2.5	55.5	14.3 (as lactate)		138
5% Dextrose in half strength oral Hartmann's solution	66	3	56	14 (as lactate)	188	
4% Dextrose and 0.18% sodium chloride	30		30		150	286
Darrow's solution	121	35	103	53 (as lactate)		313
Ringer's solution	147	4	155			
0.9% sodium chloride (isotonic, normal saline)	150		150			325
5% Dextrose					188	276

*Lancet, 1975, 1, 79

General practice management

From a consideration of all the above information and study of the contents of the commonly used replacement fluids it can be seen why the 'ideal' oral solution (Table 28) is ideal for general practice use. Table 29 details a 'mother's solution' which can be made from ingredients available in most households. If a mother can be relied upon not to make up hyperosmolar solutions this is a suitable 'general practice' replacement solution. If the mother cannot be relied upon the child should probably be treated with cooled boiled water for only a brief period: if improvement does not occur hospital admission should be considered.

Table 29   Mother's solution: practical domiciliary management of vomiting and diarrhoea. Addition of unsweetened fruit cordial will provide flavouring and a little potassium. The solution contains 90 mmol/l of sodium, 30 mmol/l of bicarbonate and 110 calories

To one litre of sterile water add:	*Equivalent in level (5 ml) teaspoonfuls*
3.5 grams domestic salt	1.0
2.5 grams baking soda (sodium bicarbonate)	¾
20 grams glucose	8 (or 4 of domestic sugar is a suitable alternative)

GUIDES TO THE PROGRESS OF THERAPY

In hospital practice the fluid balance chart (Table 27) should provide an adequate guide to the progress of therapy but other clinical signs are of value.

(1)   If fluid replacement has been too slow the blood urea level will rise, the urinary urea level will rise (in the absence of acute renal failure) and the urinary specific gravity will rise.

(2)   If there is water overload signs of heart failure may be evident including a triple rhythm, raised jugular venous pressure, pulmonary crepitations or peripheral oedema. In these circumstances one should ensure that the patient has no pre-existent intrinsic renal disease or water depletion induced renal damage. If either of these is confirmed the next 24 hours' water intake will have to be restricted to the previous 24 hours' total water output plus the estimated insensible loss. In rapidly changing situations the water 'budgeting period' should be reduced to 6 hours.

(3)   In infants water overload may be suspected if the periorbital tissue becomes swollen or signs of heart failure occur − an increase in liver size is especially common in infantile heart failure.

(4) An increase in body weight above the pre-illness normal suggests water overload or excessive fluid retention.

RE-INTRODUCTION OF NORMAL FEEDING

Adults should have a gradual transfer to a normal diet after symptoms have resolved.

A commonly used regimen to re-introduce infant feeds once diarrhoea has stopped is to give ¼ strength feeds for 12–24 hours, then ½ strength feeds for 12–24 hours and then to resume full strength feeds if diarrhoea does not recur. If diarrhoea does recur during the re-introduction of infant mild feeds one should revert to the previous milk or fluid concentration and later try again with the 'failed' concentration. If relapse recurs yet again, consider the possibility of (1) either secondary lactase deficiency causing lactose intolerance and use lactose-free milks (for example Galactomin), or (2) cow's milk protein intolerance for which soya bean milk may be used (for example Velactin or ProSorbee): altered cow's milk can also be used (for example Nutramigen).

Lactase deficiency can be confirmed by the lack of rise in blood glucose after an oral lactose load and by enzyme assay of small bowel biopsy enzyme levels. In lactase deficiency the stools are acidic and contain reducing substances which can be detected using 'Clinitest' tablets. The breath hydrogen content can also be measured after an oral lactose load.

Most children with cow's milk protein intolerance also have a lactase deficiency.

Very rarely temporary intestinal intolerance of glucose occurs and oral glucose has to be discontinued and intravenous therapy instituted.

In any prolonged diarrhoea the need for vitamin supplements should not be forgotten.

Suggested further reading

Higginson, A.G. (1979). Travellers' Diarrhoea. *Practitioner*, **223**, 529

Palmer, D.L., Koster, F.T., Islam, A.F.M.R., Rabman, A.S.M.M. and Sack, R.B. (1977). Comparison of sucrose and glucose in the oral electrolyte therapy of cholera and other severe diarrhoeas. *N. Engl. J. Med.*, **297**, 1107

Pierce, N.F. and Hirschhorn, N. (1977). Oral fluid – a simple weapon against dehydration in diarrhoea. *WHO Chron.*, **31**, 87

14
Prevention of infectious diseases

INTRODUCTION

In principle there are three main ways to prevent infectious diseases (Table 30). In terms of infectious diseases pre-exposure prevention of

Table 30 The three main ways to prevent infectious diseases

Control or eliminate the source of infection	Early diagnosis and treatment of infections, contact tracing, health education, provision of safe sewage disposal and an uncontaminated water supply, elimination of vectors, import and travel restrictions on animals, sterilization, disinfection or pasteurization procedures
Break the chain of disease transmission	All the above plus appropriate isolation of patients, washing of hands
Increase resistance to infection, either of individuals or of populations	Avoidance of malnutrition; immunization and in certain situations the use of prophylactic drugs

infection is largely dependent on immunization (defined as the act of making an individual less susceptible to an illness that may affect others).

For immunization against a disease to be worthwhile the disease must be of justifiable frequency and severity and should not be easily treatable.

Immunization may be achieved by the administration of preformed antibody, by administration of antigenically similar but less pathogenic organisms or by vaccination with killed, attenuated or otherwise modified organisms. If a disease causes major manifestations by means of toxin production, immunization may be achieved by giving an inactivated preparation of the toxin (a toxoid). An ideal immunizing preparation should promote long lasting immunity to a particular disease, it should be safe, stable and store well. It should preferably be cheap.

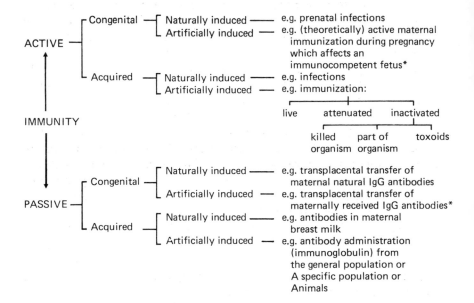

Figure 48   A classification of immune responses: these may be modified by immunodepression or immunostimulation (transfer factor or levamisole etc.).
*Most fetuses are not fully immunocompetent, †IgG alone can cross the placenta

PRODUCTION OF IMMUNITY (Figure 48)

Active immunity

This is immunity produced *by a host* in response to antigenic challenge from killed, attenuated or modified organisms or their toxins. It usually takes at least 1 week for active immunity to be stimulated by antigenic challenge.

Live vaccines function in an antigenically similar fashion to the natural 'wild' infection and usually evoke the full range of 'natural' immunological responses, including the production of local (IgA) immunity if the vaccine is given by the same route as the natural infection. In general an interval of 3 weeks or more should separate administration of live vaccines so that stimulation of non-specific immunity does not impair the host response to a second live vaccine given within this period. Recent studies have shown that certain live vaccines can be given *simultaneously* with adequate production of immunity. In general live vaccines produce greater immunity than killed virus vaccines.

Attenuated vaccines such as Sabin (polio) and BCG (tuberculosis) consist of live organisms that have been weakened by repeated culturing. Whilst they elicit an immune response to protect against subsequent challenge with 'wild' organisms, the attenuated organism may very rarely revert to a virulent state or possibly cause an illness similar to that produced by the 'wild' organism. In theory at least this latter possibility would be more likely to occur in patients immunodeficient in some way.

Save for exceptional circumstances live vaccines should not be given to vulnerable patients such as the immunosuppressed, the pregnant, those on steroid therapy or those receiving radiotherapy. In such patients inactivated vaccines should be used if available (for example administration of Salk rather than Sabin polio vaccine). If vaccination with a live vaccine is unavoidable it may be possible to give the live vaccine at the same time as the appropriate antibody to the vaccine: the vaccine replicates at the site of inoculation causing the host to mount an immune response with the administered antibody (predominantly IgG) preventing further spread of the infection. An example of this is smallpox vaccination in the vulnerable patient with simultaneous administration of anti-vaccinial antibody.

Inactivated vaccines consist of either suitable preparations of killed organisms or, alternatively, antigenically relevant parts of an organism may be given in which the immunity stimulating antigens can be presented without other constituents of the organism.

Immunity from killed virus vaccines is often a brief duration and persons at risk have to be vaccinated repeatedly — possibly leading to allergic reactions caused by continued exposure to foreign proteins.

Passive immunity

This is acquired from products, usually antibodies, derived from another host. Although effective immediately after administration such immunity is frequently short lasting because the recipient recognizes the administered antibody as a foreign protein which is then progressively eliminated.

Antibody obtained from the general population (pooled human immunoglobulin/normal human immunoglobulin) will protect against

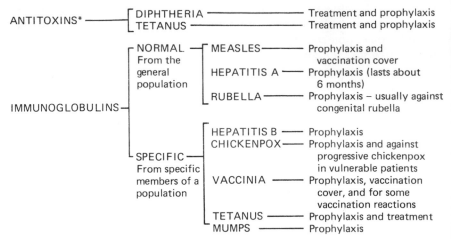

Figure 49 Currently favoured therapeutic immunoglobulins and antitoxins. *Botulism and gas.gangrene antitoxins are available: the former is useful but the latter is of uncertain efficacy

certain diseases common in that population (Figure 49). Antibody obtained from *specific* populations (such as those recently convalescent from, or recently vaccinated against, certain diseases) will contain high concentrations of the particular antibody (hyperimmune globulin). Specific antibody may similarly be obtained from animals recently infected with, or vaccinated against, certain diseases. However, these antibodies may well elicit marked 'allergic' responses from recipient humans, especially if repeated doses have to be given.

In general terms pre-exposure or immediate post-exposure administration of antibody is ideal: administration once an infecting organism is well established may not be effective and may precipitate immune mediated reactions.

Congenital immunity

Immunity is acquired by a fetus *in utero*. The fetus acquires about 6 months protection to most of the diseases for which the mother has circulating antibody by passage of maternal IgG across the placenta: thus most children less than 6 months old are protected against common infectious diseases such as measles and chickenpox.

In certain diseases drugs may be used to prevent infection – examples include penicillin prophylaxis of rheumatic fever or endocarditis.

Table 31 Currently favoured immunizations: if immunoglobulin therapy is also possible this is detailed in the text and Figure 48. Contraindications are detailed in the text

		For whom advisable	Standard course	Routine boosts advisable
LIVE VACCINES	Measles	Routine	One dose	Not required
	Mumps	Susceptible postpubertal males	One dose	Not required
	Polio (Sabin type)	Routine	3 + 1 + 1 doses	For those at continuing risk probably every 5 years
	Rubella	11–13 year old girls	One dose	Not required
	Smallpox	Occupational risk. Travel to certain countries	One dose – if 'take' recorded	Every 3 years
	Tuberculosis	Routine in Mantoux negative patients	One dose	Not required if Mantoux positive
	Yellow fever	High risk patients	One dose	Every 10 years
VACCINES PREPARED FROM INACTIVATED BACTERIAL CELLS	Anthrax	Occupation risk patients	4 doses	Every year
	Cholera	Travellers to endemic or epidemic areas	2 doses	Every 6 months
	Typhoid (Monovalent)	Travellers to endemic or epidemic areas	2 doses	At least every 3 years
	Whooping cough	Routine	3 doses	Not required
VACCINES PREPARED FROM INACTIVATED VIRAL CELLS	Polio (Salk type)	The pregnant if vaccination advisable		
	Rabies	Pre- or post-exposure	6 doses	
TOXOID PREPARATIONS	Diphtheria	Routine	4 doses	Not usually required
	Tetanus	Routine	4 + 1 doses	Immediately after at risk situations: no more than once yearly
VARIABLE PREPARATIONS	Influenza A	Those at particular risk. Essential workers	Variable	Not applicable

247

Table 32   Routine vaccinations as offered in the United Kingdom

Vaccination	3 months	6–8 weeks later	4–6 months later	12–14 months	First school year	10–13 years	11–13 years	15–19 or on leaving school
Diphtheria	+	+	+		+			
Tetanus	+	+	+		+			+
Pertussis	+	+	+					
Polio (Sabin type)	+	+	+		+			+
Measles				+				
BCG (if Mantoux negative)						+		
Rubella							+	

ASPECTS OF SPECIFIC IMMUNIZATIONS (Tables 31 and 32)

(For specific practical details the DHSS and manufacturers' literature should be consulted.)

LIVE VACCINES

Measles

Vaccination against this relatively minor disease of childhood is particularly warranted because of the small but significant proportion of sufferers who develop serious complications including chest infections, otitis media and neurological damage. As vaccination against measles is routine it is essential to have a high vaccination rate in childhood, otherwise those remaining unvaccinated will be vulnerable at a later age – when measles may be more inconvenient.

Routine measles vaccination is offered at 12–14 months and with appropriate live vaccines the protection rate* is about 85%.

Mild complications of vaccination are common: a mild reaction with malaise, fever and a rash may occur 5–10 days after vaccination.

Apart from standard contraindications to vaccination with live vaccines there are few contraindications: patients with untreated active tuberculosis or allergy to egg, polymyxin or neomycin should not be vaccinated. It is important to immunize vulnerable populations such as malnourished children and those with chronic diseases such as cystic fibrosis or heart disease.

*The protection rate is:

$$\frac{\text{attack rate in unvaccinated minus attack rate in vaccinated}}{\text{attack rate in unvaccinated}} \times \frac{100}{1}$$

Prevention of infectious diseases

Administration of normal immunoglobulin if given early enough is effective as a prophylactic measure and is limited to those in whom an attack of measles must be prevented. Vulnerable patients may be vaccinated with immunoglobulin cover.

It is of note that measles vaccination prevents more cases of measles encephalitis than it causes and the chance of developing subacute sclerosing panencephalitis is less than in a natural infection with measles.

Mumps

Vaccination with a live attenuated vaccine usually confers lifelong immunity. It is usually offered to susceptible post-pubertal males who have a 20% chance of developing orchitis if they have mumps.

Polio (Sabin)

This orally administered vaccine produces circulating antibody and also local immunity in the gut (mostly IgA mediated). There are three types of vaccine virus (corresponding to the three main types of polio virus) and these three vaccine viruses are given together on three separate occasions so that immunity to all three types of 'wild' virus can be ensured.

An outbreak of polio can be contained by immediate vaccination of encircling contacts (even before vaccine-elicited antibodies are available for defence); replication in the gut of the vaccine virus interferes with replication of a subsequent 'wild' virus infection.

As there is a minute risk that the vaccine virus may revert to a virulent state it has been advised that parents whose immunity may have waned should receive a booster dose of vaccine whenever their children are vaccinated.

Vaccination of immigrants is important as is vaccination of travellers to areas outside Northern Europe, North America, Australia and New Zealand. A pregnant woman travelling to a developing country should receive (Salk) killed vaccine unless she has to travel immediately to uncivilized areas of developing countries – in which case live vaccine would be appropriate.

The following groups of patients should *not* receive live (Sabin) vaccination: the unhealthy, those with intercurrent illnesses, those with diarrhoea, patients with hypogammaglobulinaemia, those who are immunosuppressed or on steroid therapy and patients allergic to penicillin, neomycin, streptomycin or polymixin.

Rubella (German measles)

Rubella is commonly a trivial illness, but about 15–20% of women of child-bearing age are susceptible and are thus at risk of producing a child damaged by intrauterine rubella if they are infected in pregnancy. The earlier in pregnancy the infection the greater the risk of fetal damage.

A history of a previous attack of rubella does *not* signify immunity (the clinical diagnosis is often wrong), and does *not* signify that vaccination is unnecessary. Only serological evidence should be accepted as evidence of previous rubella.

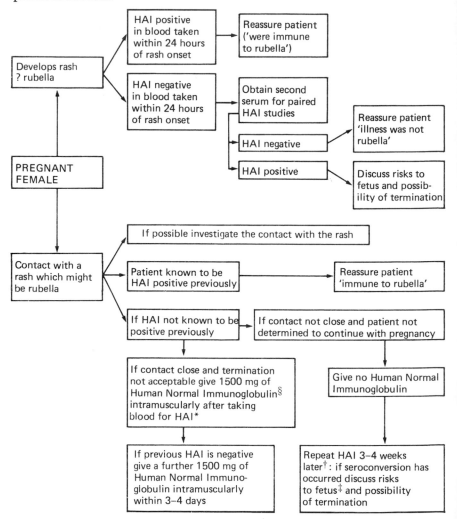

Figure 50   The suggested action to be taken if a pregnant woman is suspected of having rubella, or contact with rubella.
* Human Normal Immunoglobulin does not interfere with HAI tests to a significant degree; † Test the two serum specimens in parallel to minimize comparative laboratory error; ‡ the risks to a fetus after subclinical rubella are not known with certainty; § Passive immunization with Human Normal Immunoglobulin is of uncertain efficacy: hyperimmune serum may be better if obtainable

Immunity conferred by vaccine or 'wild' virus is not absolute and rein-
fections may occur, but the risk to a fetus *in utero* is probably low.
Although rubella vaccine is a live virus there appears to be little transmission to contacts. Vaccination of all those including males who come into
contact with large numbers of patients (some of whom may be pregnant) is
preferable: these include medical, paramedical, antenatal attendants and
ultrasound personnel.

In the United Kingdom vaccination is offered to schoolgirls between the
ages of 11 and 13 years when (it is hoped) pregnancy, an absolute contraindication to vaccination, is unlikely. Pregnant women who are vulnerable
to rubella (seronegative) should be offered vaccination shortly after
delivery: they should not allow themselves to be at risk of further
pregnancy for at least 3 months. Reactions to vaccination are usually mild,
possibly consisting of mild fever, rash, lymphadenopathy, arthralgia or
arthritis.

The use of immunoglobulin in pregnant women exposed to rubella is
detailed in Figure 50. Specific high-titre immunoglobulin in high dosage
has been shown to prevent viraemia in rubella infections and thus one
presumes that a fetus in utero would not be infected.

Smallpox

The global eradication of smallpox (*Variola major* and *minor*) is a major
triumph for the World Health Organization. Eradication was achieved by
quarantine of infected patients, rapid tracing of relevant contacts followed
by immunization, surveillance and quarantine when indicated – not by
mass vaccination. In future only certain at-risk workers will require
vaccination, but vaccination at the time of writing is still required for
travel to some countries. The International Certificate of Vaccination is
valid (for 3 years) 8 days after primary vaccination.

The origins of the live virus used for vaccination are uncertain as it differs
from both cowpox and smallpox. About 7 days after a primary vaccination
a major reaction ('a take') may occur – a typical Jennerian vesicle. A major
reaction after secondary vaccination is a vesicle, or pustule, or an area of
definite palpable induration or congestion surrounding a central lesion
which may be the seat of an ulcer. Vaccination immediately after exposure
to smallpox does offer protection, as immunity to vaccinia (and thus
smallpox) develops more rapidly than the pathogenic potential of smallpox
infection. The drug methisazone may also be effective as protective
therapy post-exposure.

Antivaccinial immunoglobulin can be used prophylactically in contacts
especially if they present too late for vaccination to be reliably prevent-
ative, and also antivaccinial immunoglobulin can be used at the time of vaccination in patients who possess relative contraindications to vaccination.

If vaccination for travel has to be performed with the minimum of delay smallpox vaccination and yellow fever vaccine can be given simultaneously − but as yellow fever vaccine has to be given at a designated centre the patient should be sent to a centre that will do both (or the smallpox vaccination should be given 'minutes' before the appointment for yellow fever vaccination).

Patients in whom vaccination is contraindicated include those with hypogammaglobulinaemia, lymphoma, leukaemia, the pregnant, the eczematous or those receiving steroid therapy. It is safer to avoid vaccinating children less than 1 year of age as the complication rate tends to be higher. A point not to be forgotten is that vaccinia is infectious and vaccinated patients should not come into contact with vulnerable patients.

Tuberculosis

Vaccination is with a live vaccine − Bacille·Calmette-Guérin (BCG) − derived from a bovine mycobacteria. In the United Kingdom it is usually offered routinely to tuberculin negative 10−13 year olds.

Ideally all those working in crowded conditions, immigrants and their children, and all medical and paramedical staff should be known to be tuberculin positive: this usually, but not always, indicates immunity to tuberculosis. If members of these groups are tuberculin negative they should receive BCG and be subsequently re-tested to ensure conversion to tuberculin positivity.

BCG need not be given to tuberculin positive patients and it should not be given to immunologically vulnerable patients, to patients currently suffering from any infectious disease, or to those on steroids or immunosuppressive therapy.

If a person known to be tuberculin negative is exposed to tuberculosis and becomes tuberculin positive he may be given isoniazid alone (to help him combat the presumed infection).

The Mantoux test is a test of cutaneous sensitivity to tuberculoprotein: a preparation (tuberculin) of tuberculoprotein given either as old tuberculin (OT) or as stabilized purified protein derivative (PPD) is injected intradermally and the skin induration elicited is recorded 48−72 hours later. One TU (equivalent to 1 : 10 000 OT) is given initially and the concentration progressively increased if there was no reaction to the previous concentration. Palpable *induration* (*not just erythema*) of over 10 mm 48 hours after administration of 5 TU is a positive result, which indicates either previous exposure to mycobacteria (not necessarily *Myco. tuberculosis*) or the presence of an active mycobacterial infection.

A negative test, up to a concentration of 250 TU (1 : 100 OT) is usually taken to indicate a lack of hypersensitivity to tuberculoprotein: this may be associated with a lack of previous infection with mycobacteria (including

BCG) or due to various 'immunologically paralysing' situations such as overwhelming tuberculosis, measles, infectious mononucleosis, sarcoidosis, steroid therapy, or in some patients with leprosy. A negative Mantoux test does *not* exclude a diagnosis of tuberculosis, and indeed in miliary tuberculosis a negative Mantoux test in a person who would be expected to be Mantoux positive may be a valuable clue.

The Tine and Heaf tests are alternative techniques used to assess cutaneous tuberculoprotein sensitivity.

Yellow fever

If properly stored vaccine is given, this vaccination is highly effective and confers long-lasting immunity. Vaccination of children less than 9 months of age should be deferred if possible because of the possibility of vaccine related encephalitis. Vaccination is best avoided in pregnancy, although the risks appear to be small, especially if vaccination is performed after the first trimester.

The International Certificate of Vaccination is valid (for 10 years) 10 days after vaccination.

VACCINES PREPARED FROM INACTIVATED BACTERIAL CELLS

Anthrax

An extract of *B. anthracis* can be used to protect patients who are occupationally exposed to anthrax.

Cholera

Cholera vaccine is a killed vibrio vaccine: it is of limited value and lasts for 3–6 months. The main defence against cholera is good medical advice – travellers to affected areas should be fastidious regarding pure water ingestion. They should avoid eating food obtained from street stalls, green salads (as the preparation may be suspect) and fruits which cannot be peeled.

The International Certificate of Vaccination is valid (for 6 months) 6 days after primary vaccination. The certificate is valid immediately after revaccination.

Typhoid (and paratyphoid)

These are often combined in the TAB vaccination (typhoid, paratyphoid A and B) which contains killed organisms. Only the typhoid component is of unequivocal efficacy and thus is often given alone as monovalent (typhoid only) vaccine to travellers outside Northern Europe, North America, Australia and New Zealand.

The family and other close contacts of a proven case of typhoid should also be offered vaccination.

Paratyphoid A is usually acquired in the Balkans or in India and protection afforded by vaccination is 'possibly useful'. Paratyphoid B vaccination appears to offer little protection.

Whooping cough

Although the need for vaccination and the incidence of vaccine related complications have been vigorously disputed it now appears that the total hazards of whooping cough are greater than the total risks of vaccination.

The age at which vaccination should be given has also been a subject of controversy. Whilst children less than 6 months of age are most at risk from an attack of whooping cough there is only slight evidence that vaccination is effective if given in the first few months of life, and one study noted reactions to vaccination to be greater in babies less than 6 months of age.

Current British practice is to immunize children at 3 months of age unless they have had whooping cough: this course of vaccination will protect a child during part of its maximum risk period and will probably prevent the child from bringing the infection home to younger siblings in the future.

As no vaccination offers 100% protection it is to be expected that a small proportion of those immunized against whooping cough will contract the disease: this fact does not invalidate the desirability of mass vaccination.

Mild reactions to vaccination are not uncommon and consist of feverishness, irritability or fretfulness. Major reactions are uncommon and include persistent screaming, collapse, convulsions and encephalopathy.

Conventionally accepted contraindications to vaccination include:

(1) Current illness of any sort.
(2) Severe local or general reactions to a preceding dose of vaccine.
(3) Seizures or convulsions, or cerebral irritation in the neonatal period.
(4) Neurological defects.
(5) A family history of epilepsy or any other central nervous system disease.

In theory at least prophylactic administration of certain antibacterial drugs (including co-trimoxazole) would offer a degree of protection if given to close contacts of a patient with whooping cough.

VACCINES PREPARED FROM INACTIVATED VIRAL CELLS

Polio (Salk)

Although not currently favoured in Britain this vaccination has been used successfully elsewhere. In Britain it is mainly used for vaccination in pregnancy, for those on steroid therapy, and for some patients with chronic intestinal dysfunction.

Rabies

Pre-exposure vaccination should be offered to those at particular risk. Post-exposure vaccination after treatment of the wound must be given to all those, *including those previously vaccinated*, who are bitten by an animal known or suspected to be rabid. An inactivated vaccine obtained from human diploid fibroblasts is given on days 0, 3, 7, 14, 30 and 90 post-exposure. Antirabies serum is also given both around the wound and intra-muscularly. The World Health Organization recommendations should be followed.

Table 33   The Schick test: if diphtheria is a possible diagnosis this test is irrelevant. Antitoxin and antibacterial therapy should be given without delay

Right Forearm
Toxoid

Left Forearm
Toxin

Intradermal
Injection

72-96 hours later

		Meaning	
Positive	No reaction	Susceptive to diphtheria toxin	A reddish area 1 cm or more in diameter: later fades to leave an area of brownish pigmentation
Negative	No reaction	Not susceptible to diphtheria toxin	No reaction
Pseudo-negative	Early transient reaction due to allergy, but fades by 72–96 hours	If both fade at the same rate the patient is not susceptible to diphtheria toxin, but is allergic to another bacterial protein	Early transient reaction due to allergy, but fades by 72–96 hours
Pseudo-positive	Early transient reaction	Allergic to bacterial proteins, probably not susceptible to diphtheria toxin	Early transient reaction due to allergy, but reaction persists

TOXOID PREPARATIONS

Diphtheria

Mass immunization with toxoid has been responsible for the almost complete disappearance of diphtheria in Britain.

There are few side effects related to immunization in infancy. In adults reactions may occur and therefore before primary immunization (or administration of reinforcing doses) to those over 10 years of age Schick testing should be undertaken (Table 33). If adults are vulnerable (Schick positive) immunization, if indicated, may be given with a reduced dose of toxoid as this is associated with fewer reactions than a full dose: it is probably less efficacious. The small amount of toxoid in a Schick test itself confers a minor degree of immunity.

Diphtheria antitoxin should be given immediately a clinical diagnosis of diphtheria is made. This hopefully will neutralize circulating (unfixed) toxin. Antibacterial therapy should also be given.

Tetanus

Tetanus is an unusual for an 'antigenically stable' infectious disease in that an attack does *not* confer immunity and therefore immunization with toxoid should *always* follow recovery from an acute attack.

After a basic course of immunization has been completed a reinforcing dose of toxoid at, or very soon after, the time of a possible tetanus exposure will boost the patient's own circulating antitoxin. Specific human anti-tetanus immunoglobulin is usually given for wounds sustained more than 6 hours previously, wounds contaminated with soil or manure, devitalized wounds and puncture wounds. Such wounds should be thoroughly cleaned, and devitalized tissue or foreign material should be removed. Prophylactic antibacterial therapy should be considered in addition to toxoid administration or immunoglobulin administration.

VARIABLE PREPARATIONS

Influenza A

Vaccines consisting of modified live virus, killed virus and fragments of virus are available. Each is of variable efficacy depending on the particular strains of virus prevalent at a particular time. The vaccines have to be updated to retain relevance to the current strains because antigenic drifts and antigenic shifts may render previous vaccines useless. The drug amantidine may be used prophylactically in high risk patients.

Immunizations under development are detailed in Table 34. Polyvalent pneumococcal vaccine is now available commercially and, at the time of writing, is still being evaluated.

Table 34 Immunizations under development

Imminent	In the future
Vibrio cholerae toxoid	Cytomegalovirus
Haemophilus influenzae type B	*Escherichia coli*
Strep. pneumoniae*	Hepatitis A
Neisseria meningitidis	Hepatitis B
	Malaria
	Pseudomonas

*Now available especially for patients with sickle cell disease or post splenectomy.

IMMUNIZATIONS FOR TRAVEL TO TROPICAL AREAS

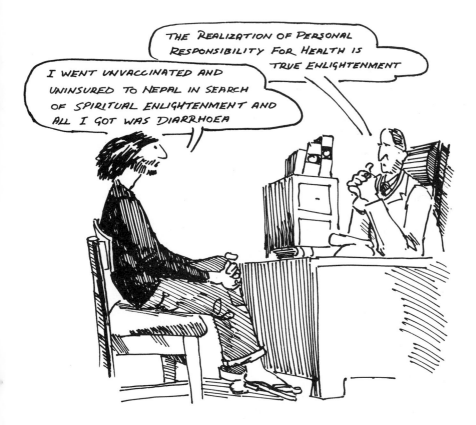

Table 35 details general advice which should be given to travellers.

Table 35   General advice for travellers to the Tropics

Dangers	Remedies
Illness	Medical insurance
Fluid intake too low	Ensure good intake
Food intake too low	Eat well
Salt intake too low	Add additional salt to food when possible
Over-exposure to the sun	Appropriate clothing
Over-exposure to *cold* (at night)	Supplementary warm clothing
Over-exposure to insects	Repellents, mosquito netting at nights
Over-exposure to sand	Appropriate clothing and goggles
Contaminated water*	Sterilizing tablets, filters, boiling of water, no swimming in natural water in Schistosomiasis areas
Contaminated food*	Avoid raw shellfish, cream, underdone meat
Contaminated ground	Wear shoes, especially if using bush latrines

*The faecal-oral route is a common mode of 'tropical' infection transmission: both food and water may be contaminated with sewage.

The indications for immunization for travel are:

(1)   To protect the traveller against diseases.
(2)   To protect the traveller against officials who may require documentary evidence of vaccination against certain diseases.

If there is any doubt concerning vaccinations required (or acceptance of headed statements certifying the presence of a contraindication to vaccination) the relevant embassies should be consulted.

Immunization programmes should commence well before travel as should arrangements for medical insurance: the National Health Service may be relatively charitable but elsewhere medical care may be prohibitively expensive.

Table 36 details the major 'tropical' or 'subtropical' diseases against which immunization is available. The doctor will need to know the countries the patient is travelling to *and through* – deaths have occurred from malaria acquired at brief stays at airports in malarial areas. It is also important to enquire what the patient will be doing in the Tropics – field biological workers may well require additional immunization against plague, rabies and typhus for example. If a child over 3 years of age has not completed the standard immunizations of childhood (Table 32) he should be given the deficient vaccinations (omitting the pertussis component).

International Certificates of Vaccination are available for cholera, yellow fever and smallpox. On *revaccination* the certificates for each are valid immediately.

Table 36   Immunizations for travel to the Tropics: a check list of major possibilities

Hepatitis A (Normal immunoglobulin)

| International Certificates of Vaccination | Cholera Yellow fever Smallpox |

Measles (for young children)
Plague
Polio
Rabies
Tetanus
Tuberculosis (if Mantoux negative)
Typhoid (? Paratyphoid in addition)
Typhus

Plague

Plague vaccine is a killed suspension of *Yersinia pestis*. Two doses are given at an interval of 4 weeks and annually thereafter for persons at continuing risk. It is usually only given to those whose occupation brings them into contact with potentially infected wild rodents.

Typhus

Typhus vaccine is a suspension of killed epidemic and murine typhus rickettsiae. It lessens the severity and mortality of the naturally acquired infection but may not alter its incidence.

Malarial prophylaxis should not be forgotten

All travellers not indigenous to malaria endemic areas *(including babies)* should take prophylactic therapy on arrival in any malarial area (or just before to ensure that there is no intolerance to the drug given), whilst in the area, *and for at least 4 weeks after leaving the malarial area.* Table 37 details general measures to reduce exposure to malaria and Table 38 the

Table 37   Prophylaxis of malaria

Mosquito netting at night
Insecticides
Wear pyjamas
Prophylactic drugs
Vaccines (under development)

Prophylaxis may fail: always tell the patient to tell doctors that he has been in a malarial area if he becomes unwell.

Table 38   Drugs used in the prevention of malaria

Drug	Mode of action	Major toxicity	Dose Adult	Dose Children	Other points
Chloroquine base Other four aminoquinolines can be used	Kills erythrocytic schizonts.	Retinopathy at high dosage	300 mg weekly	< 1 year 25–50 mg 1–3 years 75 mg 4–6 years 100 mg 7–10 years 150 mg 11–16 years 225 mg All weekly	Resistance in some areas – notably SE Asia and S America. Safe in pregnancy
Proguanil	Primarily on asexual blood schizonts. An antifolate action	Unusual. Has a wide safety margin	100–200 mg daily	< 2 years 25–50 mg 3–6 years 50–75 mg 7–10 years 100 mg All daily	Folate resistance common in some areas
Pyrimethamine	An antifolate action	Gastrointestinal (unusual)	25–50 mg weekly	< 2 years 6.25 mg 3–10 years 12.5 mg 10 years + give adult dosage. All weekly	Folate resistance in some areas. Probably best avoided in pregnancy
Maloprim = dapsone 100 mg + pyrimethamine 12.5 mg			1 tab weekly, possibly 2 weekly	5–10 years ½ tab 10 years + 1 tab weekly	Useful when folate resistance or chloroquine resistance is known
Fansidar = sulphadoxine 500 mg + pyrimethamine 25 mg	An antifolate action	Pyrimethamine + sulphonamide effects	1 tab weekly	Consult literature	Use in pregnancy under review. Effective in chloroquine resistant areas

drugs that may be used for prophylaxis. Opinions differ as to the most appropriate drugs to be taken for various areas, but if doubt exists informed and up to date advice is available from tropical medicine centres or malaria reference laboratories.

Suggested further reading

Dick, G. (1978). *Immunization.* (London: Update Books)

Immunization against Infectious Disease. (1972). Department of Health and Social Security

Notice to Travellers. Health Protection, Sa 35. (1979). Her Majesty's Stationery Office

15
Practical procedures in infectious diseases

In infectious disease practice, lumbar puncture (LP) is indicated for elucidation of suspected infections affecting the central nervous system (CNS) or, occasionally, the peripheral nervous system. Fever with neck stiffness is the most frequent indication. The exact pathological causation of neck stiffness is uncertain but common initiating factors include meningitis, sub-arachnoid haemorrhage and raised intracranial pressure with coning.

Infections distant from the CNS may cause neck stiffness without underlying meningitis, this is known as meningismus and frequent causes include urinary tract infection or pneumonia: in such circumstances a LP has to be performed as this is the only certain way to exclude meningitis. I have found that patients with meningismus headache can often shake their head without exacerbating headache in contrast to patients with a meningitic headache, who usually refuse to perform this manoeuvre.

Occasionally orthopaedic lesions, pharyngeal infections or neck tissue infections can cause neck stiffness but these should be excluded by a careful clinical assessment.

Contraindications to LP are the presence of local back sepsis, suspected raised intracranial pressure (papilloedema can be a late sign), suspected spinal cord compression (when LP should be performed at the time of urgent myelography) and suspicion of an intracranial space occupying lesion such that withdrawal of cerebrospinal fluid (CSF) might precipitate coning. Space occupying lesions that may present with a meningitic picture include neoplasms, intracranial haemorrhages and cerebral abscess. If a meningitis may be initiating or contributing to a LP contraindication, the situation should be discussed immediately with a neurologist or a neuro-surgeon, and a decision made between the performance of a LP, a cisternal puncture, or a ventricular puncture.

It cannot be stressed too strongly that the purpose of a LP is to obtain information of value, not to complete a data base. In particular, LP should not be considered a routine investigation when dealing with unconscious patients: a grossly raised CSF glucose is no way to diagnose hyperglycaemic coma!

Technique of lumbar puncture

For some reason LP has a bad reputation amongst patients and all fully conscious patients should receive an appropriate explanation and reassurance. Sedation may be given as appropriate.

(1) *Positioning of the patient*

This is crucial to successful atraumatic 'first time' LP: thus a doctor should not delegate this responsibility.

The patient should be on a firm bed or bedboards should be inserted. For a right-handed doctor the patient should be placed on the left-hand side of the bed (as viewed from the foot of the bed)

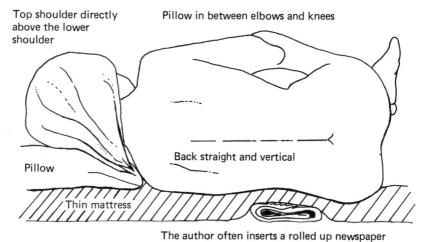

Top shoulder directly above the lower shoulder

Pillow in between elbows and knees

Back straight and vertical

Pillow

Thin mattress

The author often inserts a rolled up newspaper beneath the mattress to assist positioning

Figure 51   Positioning for lumbar puncture

with his back on the very edge of the bed such that the spine is straight in the horizontal plane and the back vertical (Figure 51). The patient's knees should be drawn symmetrically towards his chest and his head flexed downwards if, and only if, this does not cause pain. Insert a pillow beneath the head and between the knees. To achieve this position it helps if the doctor stands against the bedside and assists the flexed patient to the edge. To ensure a vertical back position, one shoulder should be directly above the other, and the transverse axis of the pelvis at right angles to the bed.

(2) *Local anaesthesia*

The adult spinal cord ends at the L1−2 level: the safest place for LP is at the L3−4 level which is usually just caudal to a line joining the anterior superior iliac spines.

I usually inject 1−2 cc of lignocaine to raise a 1 cm skin bleb and about 1 cc of lignocaine just deep to the bleb.

Whilst the local anaesthetic is taking effect and the patient is being supervised by a nurse, a face mask can be donned, as can surgical gloves after hand washing.

(3) *Check the equipment*

The lumbar puncture pack should be opened and the contents inspected to ensure all required components are present and that these all fit together. Assemble the manometer and attach the three-way tap to the lower end, such that the calibration will be facing you when the CSF pressure is being read.

(4) *Prepare the puncture site*

Apply topical antiseptic around the LP site and place towels appropriately (Figure 52).

At this stage I check local anaesthesia with a venepuncture needle. If anaesthesia is adequate I push this needle about 0.25 cm through the skin at the proposed puncture site: this assists the later introduction of the LP needle.

(5) *Introduction of LP needle* (Figure 53)

Choose an appropriate needle (the higher the gauge number − 18, 19, 20, 21 − the smaller the bore and the less rigid the needle). I immobilize the puncture site skin by placing the index and middle fingertips of the left hand on the adjacent spines.

Ensure that the needle tip bevel is horizontal (so that ligament fibres are split and not divided) and that the needle is horizontal. Direct the needle slightly cephalad (as if aiming at the umbilicus), and, between the fingers, penetrate the skin through the previous

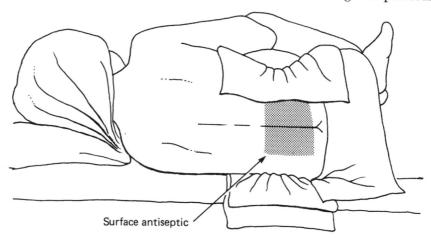

Surface antiseptic

Figure 52   Towelling up for lumbar puncture

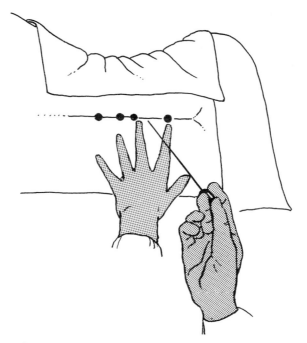

Figure 53   Insertion of lumbar puncture needle

needle tip puncture in the anaesthetized site. If the patient has meningitis it is often difficult to obtain adequate flexion of the lumbar spine and the LP needle may have to be aimed slightly more towards the head.

I usually push the needle with my right hand thumb whilst securing the needle hub between my right index and middle finger. The first resistance will be the superspinous ligament (Figure 54): after penetrating this, re-check correct needle orientation and advance the needle slowly 3.5–5 cm (in an adult) through the interspinous ligament. A little extra resistance is met when the Ligamentum flavum is reached: a little extra push (less than 5 mm) will cause a 'popping' sensation as the ligamentum flavum is penetrated and the needle enters the epidural space. Withdraw the stilette: if (as expected) CSF is not obtained, replace the stilette and advance little by little until withdrawal of the stilette reveals CSF: slight rotation of the needle may assist CSF flow if the needle tip is against a nerve root. If pain is felt in one of the patient's legs (indicating irritation of the cauda equina of that side), withdraw the needle almost to the skin and reangle it slightly towards the other side.

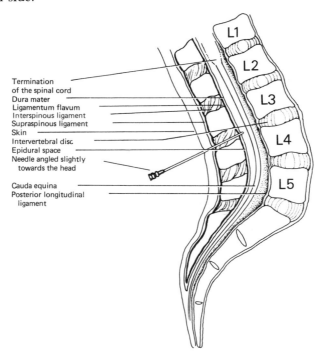

Figure 54   Anatomy of lumbar puncture

267

(6)   *CSF measurements*

Briefly replace the stilette when the CSF is obtained. Then attach the three-way tap and the attached manometer so that the CSF rises up the manometer. Check that the CSF pressure is normal and that the CSF rises and falls freely on deep respiration or gentle coughing. Then obtain three 5 ml specimens in separate bottles and a 2 ml specimen in a fluoride bottle for glucose estimation. (Ideally the blood glucose should also be measured.)

(7)   *Conclusion of LP*

After obtaining specimens withdraw the needle gently. If necessary, clean off the antiseptic and apply an appropriate covering to the puncture site: I usually use a small sterile elastoplast. Traditionally, the patient is kept flat thereafter as this seems to reduce the incidence and severity of post LP headache.

In my view intrathecal therapy should not be given at the time of an urgent LP. In an emergency situation, mistakes may be made and toxic quantities of drugs (usually penicillin) injected. I think it far safer to rely upon high dosage intravenous therapy which penetrates all areas of the CSF. The evidence that translumbar intrathecal drugs diffuse throughout the CSF is not strong.

THE CSF: ROUTINE OBSERVATIONS

In the adult the CSF is normally crystal clear, under 70–200 mm of CSF pressure and sterile on culture. It should contain no more than five white cells (all of which should be lymphocytes), less than 5.6 mmol/l glucose (not less than 0.35 : 1 of the simultaneous blood glucose level).

If the CSF is bloodstained this is usually caused by subarachnoid haemorrhage or a traumatic tap: the latter is likely if the blood swirls out only partially mixed with the CSF, if the blood clots (blood is rapidly defibrinated in the CSF and should not clot thereafter), or if bloodstaining decreases macro or microscopically with each successive 5 ml obtained. If xanthochromia is absent after the CSF has been spun down this implies that the blood has recently leaked from a vessel after a traumatic tap *or* a very recent subarachnoid haemorrhage.

If the CSF pressure is obviously very high (over 300 mmH$_2$O), withdraw the needle quickly and retain the CSF in the manometer for investigations, raise the head of the bed, place the patient supine and obtain neurological advice. Monitor the pupil size, conscious level, pulse rate and blood pressure.

If the CSF pressure is low in the absence of grossly purulent CSF emanating from a small bore needle, one should infer a blockage of CSF

Table 39 The usual cerebrospinal fluid findings in various meningitides

	White cell count Cells per mm³ Lymphocytes (L) Polymorphs (P)	Glucose (mmol/l)	Protein (g/l)	CSF Pressure (mmH₂O)	Appearance	Other points
NORMAL	Less than 5 L, No P	2.4–5.6	0.14–0.45	70–200	Clear	
PYOGENIC	400 plus, 90 % P	Less than 2	0.8–5.0 plus	Raised	Turbid	Organisms on Gram stain and on culture
LYMPHOCYTIC*						
(a) Viral	Raised: usually less than 500 ; often more than 500 in lymphocytic choriomeningitis	Usually normal or slightly low	Usually normal up to 1.0 possible	Raised	Clear or slightly hazy	No clots on standing
(b) Cryptococcal	40–400 mostly L	Often decreased	Increased	Variable	Variable	Findings depend on state of infection: CSF may be normal in early stages
(c) Leptospiral	Several 100 L	Usually normal	0.8–1.5	Slightly raised	Clear or slightly hazy	Possibly bile stained if patient is jaundiced
(d) Poliomyelitis Preparalytic	100–200 L, up to 50 % P possible	Usually normal	Usually normal	Normal or slightly increased	Clear or slightly hazy	Repeat LP in this stage usually shows a 'lymphocytic' trend
Paralytic	100–150 L	Usually normal	0.45–1.0	Slightly increased	Clear or slightly hazy	
(e) Syphilis Meningovascular	10–500 L	Usually normal	0.6–1.0	Slightly increased	Clear or slightly hazy	Serum and CSF serology positive
(f) Tubercular	50–500 L predominate	Zero–2.82	0.6–4.0	Increased	Clear or slightly hazy	Evidence of TB elsewhere? Request Ziehl–Nielsen stain and appropriate culture.

*In the early stages of most lymphocytic meningitides there may be a polymorphonuclear response in the CSF but in these instances the total count is usually low.

†The CSF: blood glucose ratio is usually 0.35 : 1. If the CSF glucose is lower then pyogenic or tuberculous meningitis is likely.

269

Table 40 The CSF findings in certain other conditions

	White cell count Cells per mm³ Lymphocytes (L) Polymorphs (P)	Glucose (mmol/l)	Protein (g/l)	CSF Pressure (mmH₂O)	Appearance	Other points
Intracerebral abscess	Variable 10–100 L predominantly	Usually normal	Slight increase 45–100	Moderate increase	Variable. Often clear	Without rupture into CSF culture may be sterile. With rupture CSF becomes pyogenic. LP is a potentially hazardous investigation
Spinal cord compression (Froin's syndrome)	Variable, usually normal. If anything L predominate	Usually normal	Increased 1–20	Low. Less than 70	Xanthochromia in 40%	CSF may spontaneously coagulate. No CSF rise and fall on coughing or respiration. Ideally do LP at time of myelography
General paralysis of the insane	40–100 L	Usually normal	Normal or increased 0.3–1.0	Often increased	Often clear	CSF serology positive
Tabes dorsalis	10–50 L	Usually normal	Normal or increased 0.3–0.8	Often normal	Often clear	CSF serology positive

outflow. Impaction of cerebellar tonsils in the foramen magnum or spinal CSF blockage can cause this: in the latter case, the CSF protein is usually raised (the Froin syndrome).

The principles here outlined apply to paediatric LP. In neonates the spinal cord terminates at the level of the third lumbar vertebra and the CSF pressure is lower than in the adult.

The classical CSF findings in various infections of the CNS are detailed in Tables 39 and 40.

FURTHER INVESTIGATIONS OF THE CSF

There are various other investigations that may be performed when the CSF gives equivocal results, a situation that may occur when antibacterial therapy has been given prior to LP.

(1) *A repeat LP* several hours later may reveal 'diagnostic trends' in cell count or biochemistry.

(2) *Counter-current immunoelectrophoresis* of the CSF can be used to demonstrate bacterial antigens, and can often provide rapid differentiation between the common agents that cause acute pyogenic meningitis including *N. meningitidis*, *Strep. pneumoniae* and *Haemophilus influenzae*. In future it is likely that this technique will be extended to differentiate between the common viral causes of meningitis.

(3) *The Limulus assay* gives rapid (60 minutes) identification of gram negative endotoxins. Essentially gelation of amoebocytes from *Limulus polyphemus* (the horseshoe crab) is produced thereby implicating gram negative bacteria as the cause of the meningitis: a negative result does not exclude a meningitis caused by other bacteria and both false positive and false negative results can occur.

(4) *CSF lactic acid quantification.* Bacterial meningitis (including tuberculous meningitis) is usually associated with a CSF lactic acid level above 4.3 mmol/l whereas in viral meningitis the level is lower.

(5) *Bromide partition test.* Serum and CSF bromide levels are measured after intravenous injection of bromide. In tuberculous meningitis the serum : CSF ratio approaches unity whereas in normals the ratio is about 1 : 3.

(6) *CSF immunoglobulins.* In the normal CSF there are only trace amounts of IgM and low concentrations of IgG and IgA. In acute pyogenic meningitis the IgM level is usually in excess of 3.0 mg/100 ml − a level a viral meningitis is unlikely to attain.

271

(7) *Gas chromatography* is a technique only available in certain centres. It characterizes trace amounts of volatile substances enabling differentiation between various meningitides.

Depending on clinical circumstances and CSF results, various other investigations can be performed including tests for syphilis, staining and culture of the CSF for fungi, and culture for viruses. In acute meningitis, tests 'peripheral' to the CNS may be indicated including blood cultures (obligatory in pyogenic meningitis), serum amylase, syphilitic serology, throat and stool cultures for viruses (significant non-CSF isolates will also be associated with diagnostic changes in serum antibody titres), paired sera antibody estimations, chest X-ray, skull X-ray, isotope brain scan, computerized axial tomography and even brain biopsy with appropriate culture and histological staining.

A SUGGESTED SCHEME FOR TAKING BLOOD FROM PATIENTS WHO HAVE HEPATITIS B*

Junior Medical Staff are often advised to 'be careful' and to 'take care' when taking blood from known hepatitis B patients or from carriers of the hepatitis B virus. Unfortunately, such advice is rarely more specific and no doubt usually causes more worry than reassurance. Additionally, it should not be forgotten that many patients may be unsuspected carriers of the hepatitis B virus and 'routine' bloodletting can never be considered to be entirely without risk of hepatitis B infection.

As there is a surprising lack of specific advice I have given the problem of safe bloodletting much thought and I think the following scheme the most sensible approach.

Preparation

(1) Write out the blood forms indicating clearly whether the patient is, or may be, hepatitis B virus positive and attach a 'Danger of Infection' label. Label all the blood bottles and work out exactly how much blood has to be taken.

(2) Place on a disposable tray a single syringe large enough to take all the blood required, the needle, a venepuncture swab, the labelled blood bottles, a pair of disposable gloves, an extra glove, a piece of cotton wool or gauze which has been drawn out into a waterwing shape, and an opened specimen bottle with a screw top (Figure 55).

(3) Obtain a suitable two-pocket self-sealing polythene bag and insert

* Reprinted from *British Medical Journal*, 1981, **282**, 1052, by kind permission of the publishers.

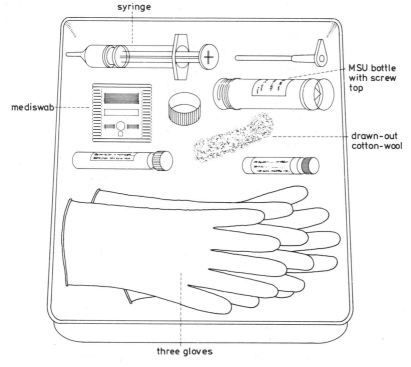

syringe

MSU bottle
with screw
top

mediswab

drawn-out
cotton-wool

three gloves

Figure 55   Arrangement of disposable tray

the blood forms into the outer packet. Attach a 'Danger of Infection' sticker to the polythene bag.

(4) Leave the polythene bag(s) in an adjacent uncontaminated position with the inner pocket gaping so that blood bottles can be placed in directly without touching the outside or entrance of the bag.

(5) Gown up ‡ and put on the pair of disposable gloves.

(6) Put a disposable paper towel beneath the venepuncture site – which should preferably be in the antecubital fossa. Place the drawn-out cotton wool on the patient's skin 1–2 in (2–5 cm) distal to the venepuncture site and at right angles to the anticipated axis of the needle.

Venepuncture

(7) Swab the puncture site and perform the venepuncture (Figure 56).

(8) After taking *only the exact amount of blood required*, release the tourniquet (if one was used it should be disposable), slide the

‡ A gowning procedure is detailed in the *Code of Practice for the Prevention of Infection in Clinical Laboratories and Post-mortem Rooms.* (HMSO, 1978). It is a moot point as to whether such recommendations should apply on the wards.

273

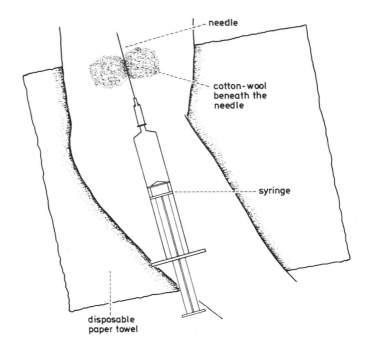

Figure 56   Position of arm for venepuncture

shaped cotton wool (or gauze) beneath the needle, advancing it until it encircles the needle at the site of venepuncture (Figure 57). Pinch the ends of the cotton wool together while pressing gently downwards on the skin.

(9)   Withdraw the syringe and needle whilst exerting very slight withdrawal traction on the syringe plunger (so that blood will not drip from the end of the needle): the cotton wool will dry the needle tip and immediately prevent any blood spillage from the venepuncture site. Then ask the patient to flex his elbow to compress the cotton wool. Never use an antiseptic swab after venepuncture – the antiseptic will sting the patient and the swab invariably becomes bloodstained.

After venepuncture

(10)   After sucking any remaining blood from the needle into the syringe, put the plastic needle sheath over the needle and remove the ensheathed needle from the syringe, placing them into the specimen bottle.

(11)   *Slowly* fill the blood bottles (to prevent foaming) and, before taking the end of the syringe out of each bottle, touch the inner

274

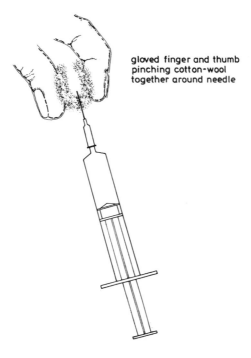

gloved finger and thumb
pinching cotton-wool
together around needle

Figure 57   Withdrawal of the needle from the arm

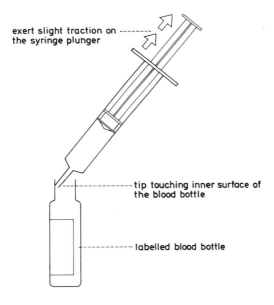

exert slight traction on --------
the syringe plunger

tip touching inner surface of
the blood bottle

labelled blood bottle

Figure 58   Withdrawal of syringe from the bottle

275

surface of the bottle with the syringe tip (so that any terminal drips enter the bottle). Then withdraw the syringe from the bottle, again exerting slight traction on the plunger (Figure 58). If the syringe has to be set down between filling blood bottles, arrange for the tip to be in the entrance of the specimen bottle on the tray.

(12) Screw on the top of each blood bottle immediately after it has been filled.

(13) Place each bottle into the appropriate gaping polythene bag.

(14) Retrieve the cotton wool and place it on the tray. Screw on the specimen bottletop.

(15) Remove the pair of gloves and gown. Wash your hands and, using the remaining disposable glove, dispose of the tray plus contents into the appropriate receptacles followed by the glove itself.

(16) Return to collect and close the self-sealing polythene bags, *touching them only on the outside.*

(17) The polythene bags should be placed within a further polythene bag or appropriate transport container. The outer polythene bag(s) should be sealed with Sellotape, *never with staples* (which would not prevent leakage and which might puncture the skin).

Although this account is rather long, in practice the whole procedure takes less than 5 minutes to complete. A simplified version serves for routine bloodletting.

Using the above technique I have eliminated blood spills and have remained negative for hepatitis B surface antigen and antibody despite occupational exposure to many hepatitis B patients.

Suggested further reading

Patten, J.P. (1972). *Lumbar puncture: indications and technique. Teach-In*, December 1972.

16

Notification of infectious diseases. Practical aspects of the treatment of infection. Tropical check-ups

Certain diseases (Table 41) should be notified to the proper officer, who is usually the Medical Officer for Environmental Health (MOEH) or the District Community Physician (DCP).

Table 41   Notifiable diseases

Acute encephalitis	Ophthalmia neonatorum
Acute meningitis*	Paratyphoid fever*
Acute poliomyelitis*	Plague*
Anthrax	Rabies
Cholera*	Relapsing fever
Diphtheria*	Scarlet fever
Dysentery (amoebic or bacillary)	Smallpox
Infective jaundice	Tetanus
Lassa fever*	Tuberculosis
Leprosy	Typhoid fever*
Leptospirosis	Typhus*
Malaria	Viral haemorrhagic fever*
Marburg disease*	Whooping cough
Measles	Yellow fever

*I would suggest that these diseases are notified on suspicion by telephone to the Proper Officer.

277

Apart from the fact that this notification attracts a small fee, the reasons for notification are:

(1)   To ensure that patients with infectious diseases are managed appropriately for the protection of the community.

(2)   To assess the present, and perhaps future, prevalence* and incidence† of certain diseases so that population management can occur.

(3)   To alert all relevant authorities so that appropriate community measures, including contact tracing, can be taken to control potential outbreaks or epidemics of disease.

(4)   To allow the efficacy of preventive measures to be monitored.

In general a clinical diagnosis suffices for notification although confirmation is obviously desirable. I would suggest that *suspicion* of certain serious diseases (marked with an asterisk in Table 41) should be initially notified by telephone so that appropriate measures can be rapidly instituted.

PRACTICAL ASPECTS OF THE TREATMENT OF INFECTION

The first point to be made is that any problem should be discussed with a relevant microbiologist, as they are usually aware of current patterns of community and hospital based infection, and can give advice concerning specimen collection and appropriate antimicrobial therapy.

Drug treatment of infection can be divided into four aspects – the patients, the possible causative organism(s), the investigatory specimens required and the drug used for treatment.

The patients

(1)   Never give a drug to a patient who does not require it: I doubt whether the tonnage of penicillin prescribed reflects accurately the true incidence of penicillin sensitive infections. If a drug is given inappropriately, serious side-effects may occur and the true diagnosis delayed or concealed.

(2)   Always check that a patient is not allergic to the prescribed drug.

(3)   Check patient compliance: this is most important when out-patients are receiving long term therapy for disorders such as tuberculosis in which poor compliance is the commonest cause of treatment failure.

*The prevalence is the number of cases of a disease present in a unit of population at a fixed point in time.

†The incidence of a disease is the number of new cases reported in an area in a defined unit of time.

The possible causative organisms

Never assume that isolation of a specific organism completely defines the aetiology of an infection. For example, a gram negative gut organism isolated from blood culture often implies large bowel pathology or a predisposing immune system abnormality (such as a leukaemia). Multiple growths of coliforms from unusual sites suggest faecal contamination.

The investigatory specimens

(1) Whenever possible obtain pretreatment specimens for bacteriological investigation. In certain infections, such as *subacute* bacterial endocarditis, it may be best to await identification and sensitivity testing of the responsible organism before starting treatment.

(2) Ensure that the specimens taken are adequate: sputum should be sputum, not saliva. If a patient cannot provide a definitive specimen (e.g. sputum in a pneumonia or urine in pyelonephritis) perform pretreatment blood cultures which may reveal the causative organism. If a bacteria is to be cultured never put the specimen into formalin, alcohol or any disinfectant.

(3) Ensure that specimens reach the laboratory in a suitably labelled container and in a suitable state for interpretation. Always state what 'informed guess' therapy has been prescribed so that the sensitivity of the organism(s) to this drug will be reported.

(4) Always obtain easily available information – a Gram stain performed on an appropriate specimen may make initial 'informed guess' therapy more informed.

The drug

(1) When prescribing an antibacterial drug consider what factors may affect its absorption: tetracyclines for example are not absorbed if given with some antacids. Some drugs are best given with food, whereas others are best given on an empty stomach. When prescribing for out-patients remember 'three times daily' does not necessarily mean '8-hourly'.

(2) In general avoid giving antibacterial drugs topically: these may or may not cure an individual patient, but can result in cutaneous sensitivity, dermatitis, or the production of resistant bacteria which may have epidemiological significance, particularly in hospital practice.

(3) There are few indications for administration of prophylactic antibacterial drugs: bacteria may become resistant to the prophylactic

antibacterial drug, the host's normal bacterial flora are disrupted and secondary (almost invariably drug resistant) bacteria have an ecological vacuum to fill. Prophylactic therapy is indicated for some group A streptococcal infections, close contacts of meningococcal infections, some wound infections, bacterial endocarditis and vulnerable contacts of tuberculosis.

(4)   Whenever possible use narrow spectrum antibacterial drugs. Broad spectrum drugs (especially if used for long periods) may strike pathogenically irrelevant bacteria a glancing blow and thereby give them a chance to develop drug resistance.

Give antibacterial drugs in adequate dosage at appropriate intervals by an appropriate route. Delayed or diminished absorption of oral drugs may occur when patients have visceral congestion due to heart failure. Similarly, patients may absorb intramuscular preparations poorly if they are hypotensive or have a poor peripheral circulation: in such patients intravenous administration is necessary.

(5)   Always give a drug by an appropriate route. Do not expect the 'magic bullet' of an antimicrobial drug to penetrate an impenetrable barrier. Certain organisms often flourish in tissues that are anoxic because of an impaired blood supply; treating such anaerobic infections with a bloodborne drug will not ensure optimal drug levels in the infected tissues. For similar reasons antibacterial therapy is often not effective against bacteria associated with foreign bodies, cavitating lesions and anatomically defective organs: surgery may be required.

(6)   Check serum concentrations of drugs with toxic side-effects (e.g. streptomycin or gentamicin). In general terms it is the 'trough' level before the next dose that reflects imminent toxicity.

(7)   Adequate serum levels may engender a false sense of security because the drug might not be reaching the 'target tissue'. For example, intramuscular or intravenous gentamicin might achieve adequate *serum levels* when used to treat neonatal meningitis, but might not produce adequate *cerebrospinal fluid levels* and supplementary intrathecal therapy may be necessary. Even then intrathecal therapy by the lumbar route does not guarantee adequate 'target tissue' levels, as some studies have shown that therapeutic levels are not achieved in the ventricles.

(8)   In general it is best not to give intravenous antibacterial drugs by constant infusion, as high peak levels are not attained (there is evidence that high peak levels are important therapeutically) and these peaks are usually best obtained with brief duration bolus injections. Additionally there are problems when administering certain drugs with commonly used infusion fluids (Table 42).

280

Table 42   Additions of drugs to infusion fluids

In general do not add any drugs to infusions containing:

Amino acid solutions	Mannitol
Dextran preparations	Plasma
Fructose	Sodium bicarbonate
Lipid preparations	Whole blood

All infusion fluids should be examined carefully to ensure absence of visible contaminants.

(9)   Whatever the route of administration the chosen drug must be given for an adequate period – most antimicrobial drugs have an exponential killing effect (Figure 58) and the microbial population has to be reduced before the host's defences can eliminate the infection without further assistance from drugs. In certain situations prolonged therapy with antibacterial drugs is mandatory to eliminate the infecting organism – in infective endocarditis for example.

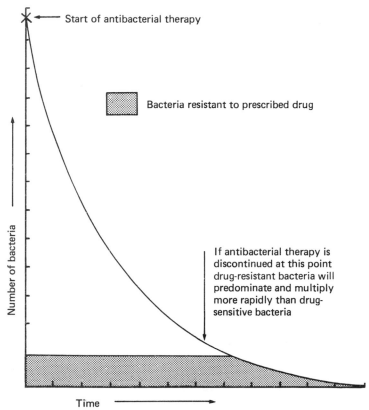

Figure 59   The exponential killing effect of antibacterial drugs on most bacteria

(10) In general give only one antibacterial drug unless there are good reasons for combination therapy. If two or more drugs are used the chances of adverse reactions are increased and certain combinations may have an antagonistic rather than an additive or synergistic effect. Drug combinations are often useful in treating infections caused by two or more invading organisms, to prevent or delay emergence of drug resistant organisms, to achieve synergism, or to enable dosage reduction of a toxic drug. Certain infections demand combination therapy (tuberculosis is an obvious example).

Adherence to the above principles will result in a more rational use of antimicrobial therapy: remember you may be 'a doctor who has everything' and you may have knowledge of the drugs to cure it – but it is necessary to select and administer the drug or drugs correctly.

TROPICAL CHECK-UPS

Asymptomatic patients who have recently returned from the tropics or the subtropics often request medical check-ups to prevent later emergence of a tropical illness. A history of the countries visited is important, but this history is useless if you have no idea where the relevant countries are or the diseases that are common there. The risk areas for some serious tropical diseases are mapped in Figures 35–42 (pages 148–153).

Questions to be asked

Where had the patient been?

When had he been there? See Table 10 (p. 147) for chart of relevant incubation periods.

What did the visit entail?

Was the visit entirely within civilized areas or were underdeveloped country areas visited?

What pre-visit vaccinations were given?

Was malarial prophylaxis taken adequately? (at least on arrival, whilst in, and for at least 4 weeks after leaving a malarial area). Those that did take adequate prophylaxis should be congratulated whereas those that did not should be informed of the risks they took, and be given advice regarding future trips. Both groups should be warned that a subsequent febrile illness might be malaria.

Had the patient been ill whilst abroad? If so, how long had he been ill, and what were the associated symptoms and signs? Ask if a doctor had been consulted, what diagnosis was made, how was the diagnosis confirmed, what treatment had been given, and had the treatment worked?

Had the patient had a respiratory illness? Is a chest X-ray now advisable?

Had the patient had a diarrhoeal illness? Are stool cultures for bacterial pathogens and microscopic stool examination for ova, cysts and parasites indicated?

Did the patient have jaundice or very dark urine? Are liver function tests (perhaps including HBsAg) indicated?

Were there any persisting skin problems or infections?

Were there any urinary problems, particularly haematuria? Should one exclude schistosomiasis?

Has the patient travelled through a bush area in West Africa within the 3 weeks prior to developing a febrile illness? If so think of Lassa fever and read Chapter 10.

Suggested 'routine' tropical investigations in well patients

The extent of routine investigations which should be performed on well patients who request 'a tropical check-up' is debatable, as is the financing of these investigations.

Two routine investigations are probably worthwhile:

(1)   A *full blood count* may reveal anaemia. Hookworm infection is a possibility in the absence of an obvious source of blood loss. Although the total white cell count may be within normal limits an eosinophilia (more than 400 eosinophils/mm^3) may well be caused by tropical worm infection – see Chapter 6.

(2)   *Stool examination* for parasites, ova or cysts may reveal evidence of asymptomatic worm or protozoal infection. Therapy of currently asymptomatic infections may prevent future illnesses and most patients are grateful for the post-treatment feeling of inner cleanliness.

In my opinion all travellers who request a routine check-up should be asked if they would like a routine test for VD – most will not, but some will be grateful for this initiative.

Suggested further reading

Benenson, A.S. (1975). *Control of communicable diseases in man.* American Public Health Association.

Index

285